OTHER BOOKS IN THE YOGA MINIBOOK SERIES

The Yoga Minibook for Longevity
The Yoga Minibook for Stress Relief
The Yoga Minibook for Weight Loss

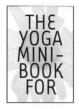

THE
YOGA
MINI-
BOOK
FOR

Energy and Strength

A Specialized Program for a Stronger, High-Energy You

ELAINE GAVALAS

Illustrations by Nelle Davis

A Fireside Book · Published by Simon & Schuster · New York London Toronto Sydney Singapore

FIRESIDE
Rockefeller Center
1230 Avenue of the Americas
New York, NY 10020

Copyright © 2003 by Elaine Gavalas
Illustrations copyright © 2003 by Nelle Davis

FIRESIDE and colophon are registered trademarks of Simon & Schuster, Inc.

For information regarding special discounts for bulk purchases, please contact
Simon & Schuster Special Sales at 1-800-456-6798 or business@simonandschuster.com

Designed by Chris Welch

Manufactured in the United States of America

3   5   7   9   10   8   6   4   2

Library of Congress Cataloging-in-Publication Data
Gavalas, Elaine.
The yoga minibook for energy and strength : a specialized program for a stronger,
high-energy you / Elaine Gavalas ; illustrations by Nelle Davis.
        p.   cm.
"A Fireside book."
Includes index.
1. Yoga.   2. Physical fitness.   3. Vitality.
I. Title: Energy and Strength.   II. Title.
        RA781.7 .G377   2003
613.7'046—dc21   2002030962

ISBN 0-7432-2700-X

DISCLAIMER

For my soul sister, Lori,
a beautiful spirit on the planet

Acknowledgments

This book would not have been possible without the help and creative contributions of my husband and writing guru, Stuart Katz. His brilliant literary judgment and patient work helped me bring this text to life. I am forever grateful for his extraordinary love, friendship, and support.

I wish to offer my heartfelt thanks to all of the talented professionals at Simon & Schuster Trade Paperbacks for producing my yoga minibook series, with special thanks to Trish Todd, for providing me with the opportunity to write the books; to my editor, Lisa Considine, for her expertise and sage guidance; and to Anne Bartholomew, Martha Schwartz, and Janet Fletcher, for their invaluable assistance.

I also wish to extend my deepest gratitude and appreciation to my literary agent, Michael Psaltis (and the Ethan Ellenberg Literary

Agency), for his wise counsel, encouragement, and support of my yoga books from the beginning.

I especially wish to thank Nelle Davis, who brought the yoga poses alive with her wonderful illustrations.

I am truly grateful to my parents-in-law, Ethel Katz Regolini and Leo Regolini, and my uncles, Arthur Vozeolas and Henry Kane, for their wisdom, help, and guidance.

Finally, many thanks to my yoga teachers (with special gratitude to Ram Dass and Bhagavan Das), and to you, dear reader. May yoga bring you lasting health, happiness, peace, longevity, freedom, and bliss. *Om shanthi* with love.

Contents

THE
YOGA
MINI-
BOOK
FOR

Energy and Strength

chapter 1

Understanding Yoga

Would you like to feel more energized and enjoy new levels of stamina? The demands of our nonstop society have made a lack of energy a widespread problem. At one time or another we all face days filled with far too much to do and too little energy to do it. What can you do to regain your vitality and reinvigorate your entire being?

You hold the answers to that question in your hands. I've written *The Yoga Minibook for Energy and Strength* for all of you who are run-down and out of shape and feel tired way too often. By following the yoga program described in this book, you can revitalize and strengthen your body, mind, and spirit. Yoga for Energy and Strength incorporates various yoga traditions, including hatha yoga, chakra yoga, power yoga, and Ayurveda, to create personalized, highly effective, and time-efficient workouts. It includes yoga exercises that use the body's own weight (and light hand weights) to help you build muscle strength. In addition, you'll find self-massage, breathing, and meditation practices to enhance your physical and mental energy.

Exercise fads continue to come and go, but after more than five thousand years, the practice of yoga is still with us—and more popular than ever. It offers a positive change in lifestyle, in which increased vitality, strength, stamina, and physical and mental well-being are natural by-products of enjoyable exercise.

The Yoga for Your Body Type Workouts in Chapter 3 feature *vinyasa* (a continuous flow of yoga poses) programs for the full range of body types. These powerfully effective workouts will make the most of the time you devote to exercise. The individual body types described in this chapter carry different names in the ayurvedic and Western physiological traditions, but whatever you call them, identifying your type and tailoring your yoga practice to it will have a powerful effect. In fact, it's the first step on the most direct path to achieving your fitness goals. With consistent practice, you'll enjoy new levels of energy and endurance, while improving cardiovascular fitness, reducing fat, and increasing lean muscle mass.

Yoga has long been acclaimed as a great way to improve flexibility, balance, and relaxation. But what's not as well known is that yoga can build muscle strength. The Yoga for Strength Workout in Chapter 4 combines strength training with yoga poses and includes a customized practice for your unique body type. You'll improve your functional fitness—in other words, your physical ability to meet the challenges of everyday life.

If you're feeling totally wiped out, try the Yoga for Energy Workout in Chapter 5. It includes energy-boosting yoga poses, along with breathing, meditation, and self-massage techniques that will maximize your physical and mental vitality. This yoga practice will help you accumulate *prana* (life-force energy) and efficiently circulate it throughout your body. You'll soon build a supply of prana life-force energy from which you can draw during times of need.

Tune up your energy centers with the Chakra Yoga Workout in Chapter 6. Practicing yoga poses, mantras, and meditations that correspond to each chakra is better than taking energy vitamins. This chapter's yoga workout helps prevent and eliminate chakra energy imbalances and blockages. With regular practice you'll increase your physical and mental well-being, enhance your vitality, and ultimately expand your consciousness.

If you're suffering from persistent fatigue, recovering from an illness, or you're a newcomer to yoga, the Yoga Basics and Relieve-Fatigue Workout outlined in Chapters 2 and 7 will help you to gently build your strength, stamina, and confidence without injury or strain.

Over the years, I've studied and practiced many hatha yoga styles, such as Integral, Iyengar, ashtanga vinyasa, kundalini, mantra, raja, and tantra, and have been especially interested in yoga's therapeutic applications. I've observed individuals and groups practicing yoga, and I've seen its power to help people relieve stress and lose weight while they increase their energy, strength, and longevity. I've had an opportunity to apply yoga techniques to help people achieve their wellness goals, and observed spectacular results. I've written my yoga minibook series—the first four being *The Yoga Minibook for Weight Loss, The Yoga Minibook for Stress Relief, The Yoga Minibook for Longevity,* and *The Yoga Minibook for Energy and Strength*—as self-help guides in response to people's many fitness, wellness, and diet problems, questions, and concerns.

My greatest wish is to share with you the many wonderful benefits yoga practice has given to me and the individuals I've assisted over the years. Whether you're looking to boost your energy, lose weight, relieve stress, or find the fountain of youth, I've created a yoga book for you.

But before we dive in, a little background.

21st Century Yoga

Throughout the centuries, yoga has redefined and re-created itself to meet the needs of different eras and cultures. Yoga was barely known in the Western world until the 1960s, when the Beatles went off to India to find spiritual enlightenment with Maharishi Mahesh Yogi. Since then, yoga has evolved from a practice for hippie spiritual seekers chanting *om* with Swami Satchidananda at Woodstock in 1969 to a practice embraced by everyone from Hollywood stars striving for beautiful bodies to high-powered CEOs seeking stress relief, to baby boomers wanting to turn back the hands of time. Even United States Supreme Court Justice Sandra Day O'Connor takes a weekly yoga class. At least fifteen million Americans include some form of yoga in their fitness regimen.

Although yoga has been celebrated as the new fitness philosophy for the twenty-first century, the practice of yoga actually goes back thousands of years. Yoga originated in India and is an ancient philosophical discipline, not a religion. Originally yoga was practiced as a path to spiritual enlightenment, a way of arriving at a state of pure bliss and oneness with the universe. *Yoga* is a Sanskrit word meaning "union"; it describes the integration of body, mind, and spirit, and communion with a universal energy, the Supreme Consciousness. The practice of hatha yoga, whose exercises are familiar to many Westerners, was originally devised to strengthen the body and prepare it for the long, motionless hours of meditation.

Yoga dates back to the ancient Vedas, sacred Hindu scriptures first recorded around 2500 B.C.E. Over millennia, the yoga tradition has evolved into eight principal branches, different paths that all lead to the same goal: enlightenment.

The eight branches of yoga are called the Wheel of Yoga. They include:

Hatha Yoga (pronounced *haht-ha*), the yoga of physical discipline and bodily mastery. This is the branch of yoga most of us in the West are familiar with, and it is the one presented in this book. In hatha, enlightenment is achieved through spiritualized physical practices including asanas (postures), *pranayama* (controlled breathing) and meditation. The *Hatha Yoga Pradipika*, a fourteenth-century text, is a guide to hatha yoga.

Jhana Yoga (pronounced *gyah-nah*), the yoga of wisdom and knowledge. In jhana, enlightenment and self-realization are achieved through the teaching of nondualism, the elimination of illusion, and direct knowledge of the divine.

Bhakti Yoga (pronounced *bhuk-tee*), the path to achieve union with the divine through love and acts of devotion.

Karma Yoga (pronounced *kahr-mah*), the path of enlightenment through selfless service and actions.

Mantra Yoga (pronounced *mahn-trah*), the yoga of sacred sounds for self-awakening. A form of mantra yoga familiar to Westerners is Transcendental Meditation (TM).

Kundalini Yoga (pronounced *koon-da-lee-nee*), the activation of the latent spiritual energy stored in the body and raised along the spine to the head through the breath and movement.

Tantra Yoga (pronounced *tahn-trah*), union with all that you are, achieved by harnessing sexual energy. Although tantra yoga has become famous for some rituals that spiritualize sexuality, it is essentially a spiritual discipline of nonsexual rituals and visualizations that activate spiritual energy.

Raja Yoga (pronounced *rah-jah*)—also known as royal, classical, eight-limbed, or *ashtanga* (not to be confused with the separate ashtanga style of yoga)—yoga of the mind and mental mastery. In the second century B.C.E., the great Hindu sage Patanjali wrote down the principles of classical yoga in the *Yoga Sutras*. Patanjali describes eight steps, or "limbs," known as the Tree of Yoga. These eight limbs provide ethical guidelines for living and help along the yoga path to enlightenment.

The Tree of Yoga is composed of:

Yama (pronounced *yah-mah*), the roots of the tree, which are moral discipline and ethical restraints. These include nonviolence (*ahimsa*), truthfulness, freedom from avarice, chastity, and noncovetousness.

Niyama (pronounced *nee-yah-mah*), the trunk of the tree. It is made up of self-restraints and observances, including cleanliness, contentment, self-discipline, introspection or self-study, and devotion.

Asana (pronounced *ah-sah-nah*), the branches of the tree. It includes the postures of hatha yoga.

Pranayama (pronounced *prah-nah-yah-mah*), the leaves of the tree. It includes breath control for circulation of prana, life-force energy.

Pratyahara (pronounced *prah-tyah-hah-rah*), the bark of the tree. It includes withdrawal of the senses for meditation.

Dharana (pronounced *dah-rah-nah*), the sap. It includes concentration for meditation.

Dhyana (pronounced *dee-yah-nah*), the flower. It includes the practice of meditation.

Samadhi (pronounced *sah-mah-dhee*), the fruit. It is the state of pure consciousness, or total bliss. All of the limbs of yoga lead to samadhi.

Your Yoga Practice

Whether you're nine or ninety, you can enjoy and greatly benefit from practicing yoga. Its requirements are minimal. You need only 30 to 60 minutes each day; a nonskid mat; comfortable, nonrestrictive clothing; and a small exercise space. Turn off your phone, put on the answering machine, and let your family and friends know that you're not to be disturbed during your yoga time—unless, of course, they want to join you. You'll be able to create your own yoga energy and strength home practice by following the yoga programs presented in Chapters 2 through 7.

You'll notice that the practice workouts in this book include poses that stretch the spine in six directions. In yoga there is a saying, "You're as young as your spine." If you stretch your spine in six directions during your daily practice you will be richly rewarded with a youthful, flexible, strong back and body. The six directions (and some representative poses) are:

- Forward (Standing Forward Bend)
- Backward (Standing Backbend)
- Right side (Seated Side-to-Side Right)
- Left side (Seated Side-to-Side Left)
- Right twist (Seated Twist Right)
- Left twist (Seated Twist Left)

Yoga is a noncompetitive practice. There's no need to compete with other yogis or yoginis. Simply do the best that you can each and every time you practice. Your body will respond differently to the poses from day to day because of various factors, such as your diet, the amount of sleep you've had, and the time of day you're practicing. It is important to remember that the practice of yoga is a journey and an exploration into the nature of your self.

Practicing yoga is well worth it. If you're interested in having additional energy, strength, and stamina, resulting in radiantly good health, then this is the book for you. *Namaste!* (*Namaste* is a traditional yoga blessing that means "The divine in me bows to the divine in you.")

Your Yoga for Energy and Strength Program

The Yoga for Energy and Strength Program consists of five steps to help you revitalize your body, mind, and spirit, and get in shape in the shortest time possible. Begin with Step 1 and continue with Steps 2 through 5, according to your physical condition and capabilities. An overview of each step and workout plan follows. Detailed instructions for the workout plans can be found in Chapters 2 through 7.

Step 1: Yoga Basics and Relieve-Fatigue Workout Plan

Step 2: Yoga for Your Body Type Workout Plans

Step 3: Yoga for Strength Workout Plan

Step 4: Yoga for Energy Workout Plan

Step 5: Chakra Yoga Workout Plan

STEP 1. YOGA BASICS AND RELIEVE-FATIGUE WORKOUT PLAN

Begin with the Yoga Basics and Yoga Relief poses found in Chapters 2 and 7, and practice for 2 weeks. Do these poses for 30 minutes, 3 or 4 days a week. Each practice session includes Warm Up, postures practice, and a Cool Down/Relaxation period. Be aware that it may take you more than 2 weeks to do this routine comfortably, depending on your physical condition. If you feel comfortable and confident doing these poses, proceed to the Yoga for Your Body Type Workouts. Otherwise, stay with this program until you feel strong enough to continue. See Chapters 2 and 7 for the detailed workout.

STEP 2. YOGA FOR YOUR BODY TYPE WORKOUT PLANS

After about 2 weeks of the Yoga Basics and Relieve-Fatigue Workout, select one of the four 4-week Yoga for Your Body Type Workouts in Chapter 3—Beginner, Beginner-Intermediate, Intermediate, or Maintenance. Each practice session includes Warm Up; Sun Salutation A, B, or C; and a Cool Down/Relaxation period, customized for your unique body type. As you progress from Beginner to Maintenance over a period of 3 months and beyond, you'll build your yoga practice up from 30 to 60 minutes a day, 3 to 6 days a week, depending on your body type. See Chapter 3 for the detailed workouts.

For additional energy and strength benefits, you can incorporate the Yoga for Strength Workout (see Chapter 4), the Yoga for Energy Workout (see Chapter 5), and/or the Chakra Yoga Workout (see Chapter 6) into your practice.

1. Beginner Yoga for Your Body Type Workout Plan
Weeks 1 through 4

Start with the Beginner Yoga for Your Body Type Workout and practice Sun Salutation A as prescribed for your body type, 3 or 4 days a week for 25 to 35 minutes.

2. Beginner-Intermediate Yoga for Your Body Type Workout Plan
Weeks 1 through 4

After completing the Beginner Yoga for Your Body Type Workout, continue with the Beginner-Intermediate Yoga for Your Body Type Workout and practice Sun Salutation B as prescribed for your body type, 4 or 5 days a week for 30 to 40 minutes.

3. Intermediate Yoga for Your Body Type Workout Plan
Weeks 1 through 4

After completing the Beginner-Intermediate Yoga for Your Body Type Workout, continue with the Intermediate Yoga for Your Body Type Workout and practice Sun Salutation C as prescribed for your body type, 4, 5, or 6 days a week for 30 to 50 minutes.

4. Maintenance Yoga for Your Body Type Workout Plan
Week 1 and Beyond

After completing the Intermediate Yoga for Your Body Type Workout, continue with the Maintenance Yoga for Your Body Type Workout and practice Sun Salutation A, B, or C as prescribed for your body type, 4, 5, or 6 days a week for 30 to 50 minutes.

STEP 3. YOGA FOR STRENGTH WORKOUT PLAN

The 4-week Yoga for Strength Workout can be practiced alone or in combination with the Yoga for Your Body Type Workouts. Practice these poses according to your body type for 15 to 30 minutes a day, 2, 3, or 4 days a week. Be aware that it may take you more than 4 weeks to do this routine comfortably, depending on your physical condition. See Chapter 4 for the detailed workout.

STEP 4. YOGA FOR ENERGY WORKOUT PLAN

The 4-week Yoga for Energy Workout can be practiced alone or combined with the Yoga for Your Body Type Workouts. Do these poses for 20 to 30 minutes, 3 days a week. Be aware that it may take you more than 4 weeks to do this routine comfortably, depending on your physical condition. See Chapter 5 for the detailed workout.

STEP 5. CHAKRA YOGA WORKOUT PLAN

The 4-week Chakra Yoga Workout can be practiced alone or combined with the Yoga for Your Body Type Workouts. Do these poses for 20 to 30 minutes, 3 days a week. Be aware that it may take you more than 4 weeks to do this routine comfortably, depending on your physical condition. See Chapter 6 for the detailed workout.

chapter 2

Before You Begin

Before you begin your Yoga for Energy and Strength Program, you should think carefully and realistically about your goals, and heed the following cautions. You can then begin your energy and strength program with Step 1, the Yoga Basics and Relieve-Fatigue Workout Plan.

A Word of Caution

Yoga should never cause you pain. Due to the intense stretching in some of the yoga poses, you need to be tuned in to your body. You should be aware of and realistic about where your "edge"—the point beyond which your body can't comfortably go any further—is in each pose. Being at your edge should never cause a burning feeling of pain. As you explore each yoga pose, go slowly and cautiously, finding the point to which you can stretch safely. As you gradually become stronger and more flexible, your edge will change. You'll be able to comfortably and safely stretch further and hold the poses longer.

Before beginning any new exercise program, you should always consult your health care practitioner, especially if you have health problems or physical limitations. Also, women should be aware that practicing inverted postures, such as Supported Shoulderstand with Wall and Legs-up-the-Wall Pose, is not recommended during the first few days of menstruation. If you are pregnant, be sure to obtain clearance from your physician before beginning a hatha yoga program. There are many excellent prenatal yoga classes with certified instructors that teach specific prenatal yoga routines.

Never practice yoga poses that cause you pain or discomfort. If pain persists, be sure to consult your health care professional.

Your Energy and Strength Goals

Before beginning your yoga practice, try to be clear about your energy and strength goals. How much time are you giving yourself to reach them? Set reasonable goals and know that anything worth striving for takes time. Starting with your first yoga lesson, you'll notice a boost in your energy. However, it usually takes a minimum of 2 to 3 months of consistent yoga practice to build up healthful habits that will revitalize and strengthen your body, mind, and spirit.

It also takes a minimum of 2 to 3 months of consistent yoga exercise before changes in strength, flexibility, and body composition (less fat and more muscle) begin to appear. Depending on your physical condition when you begin this yoga program, it may even take 6 months or more before your body really starts to show results. You may want to begin a yoga journal and jot down your thoughts about how you look and feel, to help you focus on areas you would like to change.

It's a good idea to check your progress every month or two and reassess your goals. For example, after 6 weeks you may be finishing the Beginner Yoga for Your Body Type Workout (in Chapter 3). At that point, you will want to determine your progress, consider what types of physical challenges you may be experiencing, and set new energy and strength goals. Depending on these results, you may want to progress to the Beginner-Intermediate Yoga for Your Body Type Workout and incorporate the Yoga for Strength Workout, or the Yoga for Energy Workout, or the Chakra Yoga Workout into your practice.

Or you may decide to continue practicing the Beginner Yoga for Your Body Type Workout without any additional workouts for a while longer.

Please keep in mind that the Yoga for Energy and Strength Program not only consists of workouts, but it is also a lifestyle modification program designed to establish good habits to improve and protect your health and appearance. Make a daily affirmation to yourself to reach your energy and strength goals through yoga exercise and breathing and meditation practice.

Yoga Basics

An understanding of certain fundamental movements will help you to perform the yoga postures in this book correctly. The following basic yoga preparations are incorporated into many yoga postures and will help you build strength, flexibility, and proper alignment in your upper body and lower back.

The squeeze, hold, and release actions found in Shoulder Press and Squeeze and Pelvic Tilt are fundamental to yoga practice. They massage tension and stress out of a particular area while bringing fresh, oxygenated blood into the muscles and tissues. The action of lifting the sternum (see Mountain Pose, page 25) is repeated over and over again within many yoga postures.

The use of your core strength—the lifting of your abdominals for maximum support—is also essential while performing yoga postures. In yoga, this includes the *mula bandha,* or "root lock," which contracts the perineum (see Root Lock, page 29) and the *uddiyana bandha,* which contracts the abdomen (see Stomach Lift, page 30). The mula bandha and uddiyana bandha actions draw awareness to the core of your body. These contractions build a strong foundation in your body and strengthen the abdominal, pelvic, and genital muscles.

Ujjayi breathing is a classic *pranayama* (yoga breathing) technique. It can be joined with Sun Salutation asanas (see pages 51 to 84) to help link the postures together and energize your practice. After yoga practice it's important to relax deeply in a pose such as Supported Relaxation Pose (page 196) and practice Yoga Observation (page 31) for a few minutes to enhance the effectiveness of the poses and calm your mind and nervous system.

Yoga Basics and Relieve-Fatigue Workout Plan

Begin your first 2 weeks of yoga practice with the Yoga Basics poses you will find in this chapter and the Yoga Relief poses in Chapter 7. Be aware that it may take you more than 2 weeks to do this routine comfortably, depending on your physical condition. If you feel comfortable and confident doing these poses, proceed to the Yoga for Your Body Type Workouts in Chapter 3. Otherwise, stay with Weeks 1 and 2 until you feel strong enough to continue.

Week 1

Practice Schedule: Practice for 30 minutes, 3 or 4 times a week. Warm up with Yoga Basics poses, proceed to Yoga Relief poses, and then cool down with a few more Yoga Basics poses.

Warm Up:

Shoulder Press and Squeeze

Pelvic Tilt

Mountain Pose and Lifting the Sternum

Chest Expander

Yoga Relief (from Chapter 7):

Seated Forward Hang

Seated Wheel Pose

Seated Side-to-Side

Seated Twist

Seated Leg Lifts

Cool Down:

Ujjayi Breathing

Root Lock

Supported Relaxation Pose and Yoga Observation

Week 2

Practice Schedule: Practice for 30 minutes, 3 or 4 times a week. Begin with Yoga Basics poses, proceed to Yoga Relief poses, and then cool down with a few more Yoga Basics poses.

Warm Up:

Shoulder Press and Squeeze

Pelvic Tilt

Mountain Pose and Lifting the Sternum

Chest Expander

Yoga Relief—Choose either Routine 1 or Routine 2:

Routine 1:

Mountain Pose Variation

Legs-up-the-Wall Pose

Supported Bridge Pose

Modified Child's Pose with Self-Massage

Or

Routine 2:

Mountain Pose Variation

Lying Bound Angle Pose

Supported Shoulderstand with Wall

Modified Fish Pose

Cool Down:

Root Lock

Ujjayi Breathing

Stomach Lift

Supported Relaxation Pose and Yoga Observation

Yoga Basics Poses

SHOULDER PRESS AND SQUEEZE

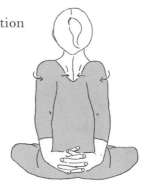

What It Does: These shoulder movements are incorporated into many yoga postures, including Chest Expander, Cobra, Downward Facing Dog, Inclined Plane, and Dolphin Headstand Preparation. The squeeze, hold, and release actions are fundamental to yoga practice, massaging tension and stress out of a particular area while bringing fresh, oxygenated blood into the muscles and tissues.

How to Do It:

1. Sit up straight on the mat with your legs crossed, arms at your sides.

2. Inhale and raise your shoulders toward your ears. Squeeze and hold for 4 counts. Exhale and release, pressing your shoulders down and away from your ears.

3. Clasp your hands behind your back. Inhale and straighten your elbows. Press your shoulders down and away from your ears. Exhale and gently squeeze your shoulder blades together. Hold for 3 counts. Release your hands.

4. Repeat.

MOUNTAIN POSE (TADASANA) AND LIFTING THE STERNUM

What It Does: The subtle but important action of lifting the sternum, or breastbone, toward the ceiling is incor-

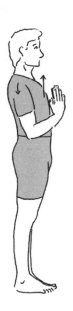

porated into many yoga postures, including Standing Backbend and Standing Bow.

How to Do It:

1. Stand in Mountain Pose: feet together, legs straight, and hands in prayer position over your heart center. Visualize a string attached to your sternum (the bone in the center of your chest).

2. Inhale and visualize the string being pulled up toward the ceiling. Feel the subtle lifting and expanding of your chest, rib cage, and sternum, lengthening the front of your body. Keep your shoulders relaxed and down, away from your ears.

3. Exhale and release.

4. Repeat.

PELVIC TILT

What It Does: These pelvic movements are incorporated into many yoga postures, including Standing Backbend, Cobra Pose, and Locust Pose with Leg Weights. The lower-back press, hold, and release actions are fundamental movements in yoga, massaging tension and stress away while bringing fresh, oxygenated blood into the muscles and tissues. It is essential to tighten the buttock muscles firmly to protect and stabilize your lower back and activate the abdominals.

How to Do It:

1. Lie on your back on the mat, knees bent and feet flat on the mat, hip-width apart. Rest your hands on your abdomen. Inhale and allow your lower back to arch naturally.

2. Exhale, tightening your buttock muscles, tilting your pelvis under, and pulling your abdomen in. Press the small of your back gently to the mat. Inhale and release.

3. Repeat.

CHEST EXPANDER

What It Does: This exercise incorporates all three movements that came before: the Shoulder Press and Squeeze, Mountain Pose and Lifting the Sternum, and Pelvic Tilt. If your shoulders and chest are tight, try clasping a towel or belt behind you while doing this exercise.

How to Do It:

1. Stand with your feet hip-width apart and clasp your hands behind your back.

2. Inhale, lifting your sternum toward the ceiling as you press your shoulders down and away from your ears. Exhale, straightening your elbows and gently squeezing your shoulder blades together. Tighten the buttock muscles, tilt the pelvis under, and pull the abdomen in.

3. Inhale, release, and relax.

UJJAYI BREATHING *(UJJAYI PRANAYAMA)*

What It Does: Ujjayi breathing is a classic pranayama (yoga breathing) technique. It is joined with Sun Salutation to help link the postures together and energize your practice.

How to Do It:

1. Keeping your lips closed, constrict the back of your throat, or glottis (the opening between the vocal chords), during inhalation

and exhalation. This produces a hissing sound, like that heard at the approach of Darth Vader.

2. If this is too difficult, try to whisper the sound *aaah* while inhaling and exhaling through your open mouth.

3. Close your lips and breathe through your nose, continuing to make the hissing or *aaah* sound at the back of your throat.

ROOT LOCK *(MULA BANDHA)*

What It Does: The *mula bandha,* or "root lock," contracts the perineum, or pelvic floor, which comprises the pubococcygeus muscles between the rectum and genitals. This draws awareness to the core of your body, builds a strong foundation in your body, and strengthens the abdominal, pelvic, and genital muscles.

How to Do It:

1. Sit on a chair or cross legged on the floor, sitting straight and tall. To visualize where your pelvic muscles are, imagine stopping the flow of your urine. Inhale, then exhale and contract these muscles, pulling up through your genital area and drawing up through your spine. Inhale and release the muscles.

2. Isolate the muscle group around your anus. Inhale, then exhale, contracting these muscles and drawing them upward. Inhale and release the muscles.

3. Now combine the two actions. Inhale, then exhale and contract the muscles of your anus and genitals at the same time. Inhale and release the muscles.

STOMACH LIFT (UDDIYANA BANDHA)

What It Does: It strengthens the abdominal muscles and keeps them flexible, and it tones and massages the abdominal organs and glands. Practice it on an empty stomach.

How to Do It:

1. Stand with your feet hip-width apart. Bend forward from the hips with your knees bent. Place your hands on your thighs above the knees for leverage. Lean the weight of your torso into your hands.

2. Exhale forcefully from your mouth. Close your mouth and bring your chin to your throat.

Hold the exhalation and pull your abdomen back toward the spine and up toward the solar plexus.

3. Hold for 2 seconds, then rhythmically pump the abdominal muscles in and out with a pull-in, release motion, 5 or more times.

4. Before the lack of oxygen becomes uncomfortable, relax the abdominals and inhale slowly. Return to an upright position.

YOGA OBSERVATION

What It Does: Yoga Observation practices "the understanding of self," *svadhyaya*, which is part of niyama, one of the eight limbs of yoga described in Patanjali's *Yoga Sutras* (see Chapter 1). This practice includes self-observation, which nurtures introspection, serenity, and cosmic connectedness, ultimately leading to a universal union with all that you are.

How to Do It:

1. Sit straight in a chair with your legs together and feet flat on the floor, or lie down in Supported Relaxation Pose (page 196). Be sure that you're comfortable and relaxed in this position.

2. Applying self-observation helps you discover and sense changes in your body and mind. For several minutes or longer, sense the

changes going on in your body externally and internally. Observe how you're feeling. How does your skin feel? Does it tingle? Is it warm? After your yoga stretches, enjoy the energy and warmth flowing to areas that were previously stiff because of fatigue or tension. Consciously try to relax any areas that still feel tense, fatigued, or painful.

3. Calmly take note of the flow of your thoughts. Is your mind restless? Do you have negative thoughts and suggestions? Quiet your mind by focusing on your breath. Center your attention on the tip of your nose. Observe the coolness of the air as it flows into your nostrils, and the warmth of the air as it flows out. Hold your attention on your breath. If your mind wanders, simply bring it back to the breath as it flows in and out of your nostrils. Be in the moment.

4. Now replace your negative thoughts with positive suggestions, such as uplifting words, affirmations, thoughts, and prayers. Breathe in love, light, energy, and healing to every cell of your body. Breathe out all negativity, darkness, tension, and fatigue. Rest your body and mind for as long as you like. Practice this simple meditation daily to nourish your body, mind, and spirit.

chapter 3

Yoga for Your Body Type

The yoga workout detailed in this chapter prescribes different vinyasas (a continuous flow of yoga poses), such as Sun Salutation, for different body types. This powerfully effective combination of yoga and body typing is the most efficient way to boost your energy and strength and to maximize the benefits of your workout time. The results, I think you'll find, are spectacular. You'll increase your strength, stamina, and flexibility; experience an incredible boost in energy; and look and feel great.

The first step is to determine your ayurvedic body type. Yoga's sister science Ayurveda is an ancient Indian healing system for the body, mind, and spirit. Ayurveda, whose name is translated as "the science of life," offers a holistic program to achieve perfect health, vitality, and energy. According to Ayurveda, imbalance manifests as disease: fatigue, sluggishness, illness, and depression are viewed as signs of a body out of balance. When ayurvedic balance is reestablished, many of these health problems diminish or clear up.

Ayurveda is based on the theory of the three *doshas*, or mind-body types, which have their own set of physical, mental, and emotional characteristics; they are *vata* (air), *pitta* (fire), and *kapha* (earth). All people and things possess elements of each dosha, but one or more of the doshas may predominate in your body and behavior. For example, you may be a vata-pitta, pitta-kapha, or vata-kapha. Your unique combination of doshas is your constitution type, or *prakruti,* which establishes your unique physical, mental, and emotional makeup. One way to achieve balance, boost energy and stamina, and develop a strong body is to identify your dosha, then make appropriate adjustments in your yoga practice and lifestyle. By determining your dosha, you can choose a yoga practice that best suits you.

In modern exercise science, physiologists classify people according to three basic body types: endomorph, mesomorph, and ectomorph. If you're familiar with those classifications, you'll quickly recognize that the three ayurvedic doshas correlate with the modern physiological types labeled endomorph, mesomorph, and ectomorph (see below). As with the doshas, people possess elements of each physiological type, but most of us are more one type than another.

When we combine the ancient wisdom of Ayurveda and modern exercise physiology, we empower ourselves and our yoga practice to achieve greater strength, stamina, and energy. By merging the body type classifications found in Ayurveda and modern physiology, we can gain greater clarity and insight into the physiological functioning of the body and what it requires in terms of exercise and yoga practice.

The three ayurvedic body types and their physiological equivalents are:

Vata/Ectomorph
Pitta/Mesomorph
Kapha/Endomorph

By knowing your predominant body type and what it requires in terms of activity level, you can tailor your yoga practice to reach your fitness goals and enjoy new levels of energy and stamina while improving your cardiovascular fitness, reducing fat, and increasing lean muscle mass.

What's Your Body Type?

The following are basic descriptions of the doshas vata, pitta, and kapha and the physiological types of ectomorph, mesomorph, and endomorph. To determine which body type is most dominant for you, make a check mark over the individual characteristics that describe you. The category with the most check marks will indicate your body type. If you have almost the same number of check marks in two or three categories, your body type is a mixture of those two or three body types.

This list of characteristics will provide an approximate indication of your dosha. An ayurvedic physician can best determine your specific dosha body type. Once you know your body type, do the yoga practice for that body type (see the Yoga for Your Body Type Workout Plans later in this chapter).

BODY TYPE: VATA/ECTOMORPH

Physical Characteristics: Thin, light-boned, angular build; hips and chest are in proportion; wiry physique; tends to be flat-chested; lacks strength and muscle tone; inflexible; quick metabolism; slow to gain weight; dry skin and hair; eats and sleeps erratically; chilly hands and feet; low ratio of muscle to fat; fat accumulates below the navel (prone to potbelly on a lean frame). Prone to chronic fatigue, osteoporosis, hyperthyroidism, and hypertension.

Mental and Emotional Characteristics: Quick mind; creates and learns quickly; forgets easily; enthusiastic; imaginative; vivacious; sensitive; unpredictable; poor sleep habits. Prone to worry, anxiety, and depression.

BODY TYPE: PITTA/MESOMORPH

Physical Characteristics: Medium-sized athletic build; well proportioned; muscular; lean; broad shoulders; thick waist; narrow hips; slender legs; blond, red, or prematurely gray hair; fair or freckled complexion; warm, ruddy, perspiring skin; good stamina; voracious appetite and tendency to overeat; tends to be warm or hot; sleeps well; eats meals quickly; apple shape when overweight; gains and loses weight easily. Prone to ulcers and digestive disorders and exercise-related injuries.

Mental and Emotional Characteristics: Confident; passionate; articulate; courageous; intelligent; ambitious; assertive; energetic; adventurous. Prone to irritability and short temper.

BODY TYPE: KAPHA/ENDOMORPH

Physical Characteristics: Large, heavy, round build; wide shoulders; voluptuous or barrel-chested; high percentage of body fat; gains weight easily primarily around the abdomen and lower body; pear shape when overweight; has trouble losing weight; builds muscle easily; excellent flexibility; thick, moist skin and lustrous hair; excellent stamina; needs more sleep than vata or pitta; eats slowly. Prone to respiratory illness, food allergies, skin problems, and obesity.

Mental and Emotional Characteristics: Forgiving; affectionate; relaxed; slow and graceful; slow to anger; calm temperament; tolerant. Prone to lethargy and procrastination.

Yoga for Your Body Type

In ashtanga-style yoga we perform vinyasas, a series of poses that follow one another in a continuous flow. *Ashtanga vinyasa* features the same poses as hatha yoga, but these poses are linked together in synchrony with the breath. Ashtanga vinyasa poses, such as those featured in Sun Salutation, are done one after another so that you're constantly moving between the poses. The result is a safe cardiovascular workout that perfectly blends flexibility, strength, and aerobic conditioning.

According to medical experts, 30 minutes of moderate activity over the course of a day, 3 times a week, will reward you with a long list of benefits, including reducing your risk of developing heart disease or dying prematurely. Moderate aerobic activities include brisk walking, stationary cycling, jogging, and ashtanga vinyasa yoga. One of the misconceptions about yoga is that it doesn't provide a cardiovascular workout. On the contrary, a vigorous ashtanga vinyasa yoga practice, such as Sun Salutation, can be just as effective as many aerobic activities in improving cardiovascular health, boosting endorphins—the "feel-good" hormones—and promoting strength, flexibility, mental clarity, and self-esteem.

All body types benefit from practicing yoga vinyasas such as Sun Salutation, but each body type requires a different level of activity to create and maintain perfect health and balance of the body, mind, and spirit.

People of a **vata/ectomorph** body type benefit from light-to-moderate exercise—exercise that isn't done to the point of exhaustion. They should work out at 50 percent of their maximum heart rate (see discussion below). Most yoga poses are calming, balancing, and grounding. Doing them helps to counter vata's agitated nature. Sun Salutation vinyasas should be performed at a slow and thoughtful pace. Other beneficial asanas include Seated Forward Hang (page 187), Child's Pose (page 138), and Easy Pose (page 173).

People of a **pitta/mesomorph** body type benefit from moderate exercise that isn't overheating. They should work out at 55 percent of their maximum heart rate. Pitta individuals also benefit from calming, quieting yoga poses to counter their fiery and aggressive tendencies. Sun Salutation vinyasas should be performed at a moderate pace and with few repetitions. Other beneficial asanas include Modified Fish Pose (page 168), and twists such as the Pose Dedicated to the Sage Marichi (page 167).

People of a **kapha/endomorph** body type benefit from daily, vigorous exercise. They should work out at 60 to 65 percent of their maximum heart rate to counter their tendencies toward lethargy and obesity. Sun Salutation vinyasas should be performed with many repetitions. Other beneficial asanas include Bridge Pose (page 137), and abdominal poses such as Boat Pose (page 114).

Your Heart Rate

1. To find your maximum heart rate (MHR), subtract your age from 220. For example, for a 20-year-old woman: $220 - 20 = 200$ beats per minute (BPM).

2. To determine your exercising heart rate according to body type, find the recommended percentage of your maximum heart rate.

- For vata/ectomorph: Find 50 percent of your maximum heart rate. For example, $200 \text{ MHR} \times 0.5 = 100 \text{ BPM}$.
- For pitta/mesomorph: Find 55 percent of your maximum heart rate. For example, $200 \text{ MHR} \times 0.55 = 110 \text{ BPM}$.
- For kapha/endomorph: Find 60 percent of your maximum heart rate. For example, $200 \text{ MHR} \times 0.6 = 120 \text{ BPM}$.

3. To check your heart rate during sustained exercise: Place your index and middle fingers on the pulse point of your opposite wrist. Using a watch with a second hand, count the pulse beats for 10 seconds. Multiply that number of beats by 6 to get your heart rate. Be sure your pulse stays within your range. Check your pulse periodically throughout your aerobic workout and immediately after finishing.

4. Always pay close attention to your body's signals of overexer-

tion, such as pounding in your chest, dizziness, faintness, profuse sweating, and an inability to carry on a normal conversation due to shortness of breath. If any of these symptoms occurs, you need to slow your pace. If symptoms persist, see your doctor.

Before You Start

- Always consult your physician before beginning a new exercise program.
- If you're just beginning a fitness program, remember to work up to the recommended frequency and duration, comfortably and gradually.
- Perform the vinyasas slowly, according to your own capacity. You should never be in pain, nor should you experience breathlessness.

Yoga for Your Body Type Workout Plans

Select one of the following four Yoga for Your Body Type Workouts to boost your energy and strength and make the most of your workout time. The vinyasas presented in this chapter include the Sun Salutation and two variations for different levels of experience. You can begin the Yoga for Your Body Type Workout after practicing the Yoga Basics and Relieve-Fatigue Workout found in Chapters 2 and 7 for 2 weeks. For additional energy and strength benefits, you can incorporate the Yoga for Strength Workout (see Chapter 4), the Yoga for Energy Workout (see Chapter 5), and/or the Chakra Yoga Workout (see Chapter 6) into your practice.

Begin with the simpler version of Sun Salutation, which will help you build the stamina, strength, and coordination necessary to practice the more challenging ones. As you progress from the Beginner to the Maintenance Workout over a period of months, you'll build your yoga practice up from 30 to 50 minutes a day, 3 to 6 days a week (depending on your body type).

While practicing the first vinyasa cycle, you may feel stiff and clumsy. By the second or third cycle, the movements will start flowing more easily and the rhythm of your breathing will become more natural.

As you practice the vinyasas, focus not only on each pose but also on the use of your breath. Breath links the postures together in vinyasa practice and energizes your aerobic exercise. During your workout, maintain deep, rhythmic breathing, synchronizing the flow of yoga postures with your inhalation and exhalation. A general guideline to follow is to inhale when doing backbends and exhale when doing forward-bending postures. See the discussion of ujjayi breathing (page 28), a classic yoga breathing technique often used during vinyasa. Ujjayi breathing should be steady and controlled.

Vinyasa yoga's full-body workout and powerful combination of stretching with movements that develop strength and balance will produce beneficial physical results within a short time. Your spine will become more supple, and tight hamstrings will begin to release, as you tone, firm, and strengthen your body.

1. BEGINNER YOGA
FOR YOUR BODY TYPE WORKOUT PLAN

After practicing the Yoga Basics and Relieve-Fatigue Workout found in Chapters 2 and 7 for 2 weeks, beginners should start with Sun Salutation A. After you've finished this 4-week Beginner plan, you can proceed to the Beginner-Intermediate Yoga for Your Body Type Workout Plan. Be aware that it may take you more than 4 weeks to do this routine comfortably, depending on your physical condition. Feel free to take as much time as you need before progressing to Beginner-Intermediate practice.

For additional energy and strength benefits, you can incorporate the Yoga for Strength Workout (see Chapter 4), the Yoga for Energy Workout (see Chapter 5), and/or the Chakra Yoga Workout (see Chapter 6) into your practice.

Weeks 1 through 4

Practice Schedule:

Vata/Ectomorph: Practice for 20 minutes, 3 days a week.

Pitta/Mesomorph: Practice for 30 minutes, 3 days a week.

Kapha/Endomorph: Practice for 35 minutes, 4 days a week.

Warm Up: Perform Sun Salutation A (page 51) once slowly, holding each posture for 5 breaths.

Sun Salutation A:

Vata/Ectomorph: Perform 4 repetitions of Sun Salutation A. Pace yourself at 50 percent of your maximum heart rate (see "Your Heart Rate," page 41).

Pitta/Mesomorph: Perform 5 repetitions of Sun Salutation A. Pace yourself at 55 percent of your maximum heart rate (see "Your Heart Rate," page 41).

Kapha/Endomorph: Perform 6 repetitions of Sun Salutation A. Pace yourself at 55 percent of your maximum heart rate (see "Your Heart Rate," page 41).

Cool Down: Perform 1 repetition of Sun Salutation A slowly, holding each posture for 5 breaths. End with 5 to 10 minutes of Supported Relaxation Pose (page 196).

2. BEGINNER–INTERMEDIATE YOGA FOR YOUR BODY TYPE WORKOUT PLAN

Once you've mastered Sun Salutation A, you can progress to Sun Salutation B (page 57). After you've finished this 4-week Beginner-Intermediate plan, you can proceed to the Intermediate Yoga for Your Body Type Workout. But be aware that it may take you more than 4 weeks to do this routine comfortably, depending on your physical condition. Feel free to take as much time as you need before progressing to Intermediate practice.

For additional energy and strength benefits, you can incorporate the Yoga for Strength Workout (see Chapter 4), the Yoga for Energy Workout (see Chapter 5), and/or the Chakra Yoga Workout (see Chapter 6) into your practice.

Weeks 1 through 4

Practice Schedule:

Vata/Ectomorph: Practice for 30 minutes, 4 days a week.

Pitta/Mesomorph: Practice for 35 minutes, 4 days a week.

Kapha/Endomorph: Practice for 40 minutes, 5 days a week.

Warm Up: Perform Sun Salutation A once slowly, holding each posture for 5 breaths.

Sun Salutation B:

Vata/Ectomorph: Perform 3 repetitions of Sun Salutation B. Pace yourself at 50 percent of your maximum heart rate (see "Your Heart Rate," page 41).

Pitta/Mesomorph: Perform 4 repetitions of Sun Salutation B. Pace yourself at 55 percent of your maximum heart rate (see "Your Heart Rate," page 41).

Kapha/Endomorph: Perform 5 or 6 repetitions of Sun Salutation B. Pace yourself at 60 percent of your maximum heart rate (see "Your Heart Rate," page 41).

Cool Down: Perform 1 repetition of Sun Salutation A slowly, holding each posture for 5 breaths. End with 5 to 10 minutes of Supported Relaxation Pose.

3. INTERMEDIATE YOGA FOR YOUR BODY TYPE WORKOUT PLAN

Once you've mastered Sun Salutations A and B, you can progress to Sun Salutation C (page 67). After you've finished this 4-week Intermediate plan, you can proceed to the Maintenance Yoga for Your Body Type Workout. But be aware that it may take you more than 4 weeks to do this routine comfortably, depending on your physical condition. Feel free to take as much time as you need before progressing to Maintenance practice.

For additional energy and strength benefits, you can incorporate the Yoga for Strength Workout (see Chapter 4), the Yoga for Energy Workout (see Chapter 5), and/or the Chakra Yoga Workout (see Chapter 6) to your practice.

Weeks 1 through 4

Practice Schedule:

Vata/Ectomorph: Practice for 30 minutes, 4 days a week.

Pitta/Mesomorph: Practice for 35 to 40 minutes, 4 days a week.

Kapha/Endomorph: Practice for 45 to 50 minutes, 5 or 6 days a week.

Warm Up: Perform Sun Salutation A once slowly, holding each posture for 5 breaths.

Sun Salutation C:

Vata/Ectomorph: Perform Sun Salutation C 2 times. Pace yourself at 50 percent of your maximum heart rate (see "Your Heart Rate," page 41).

Pitta/Mesomorph: Perform Sun Salutation C 3 times. Pace yourself at 55 percent of your maximum heart rate (see "Your Heart Rate," page 41).

Kapha/Endomorph: Perform Sun Salutation C 4 times. Pace yourself at 60 to 65 percent of your maximum heart rate (see "Your Heart Rate," page 41).

Cool Down: Perform 1 repetition of Sun Salutation A slowly, holding each posture for 5 breaths. End with 5 to 10 minutes of Supported Relaxation Pose.

4. MAINTENANCE YOGA FOR YOUR BODY TYPE WORKOUT PLAN

Congratulations! At this point, you've mastered Sun Salutations A, B, and C. I'm sure you're looking and feeling great. Follow the Maintenance Yoga Power Workout Plan to stay in shape and to continue to build and maintain your energy, strength, cardiovascular fitness, and flexibility.

For additional energy and strength benefits, you can incorporate the Yoga for Strength Workout (see Chapter 4), the Yoga for Energy Workout (see Chapter 5), and/or the Chakra Yoga Workout (see Chapter 6) into your practice.

Week 1 and Beyond

Practice Schedule:

Vata/Ectomorph: Alternate between Sun Salutations A, B, and C, practicing for 30 minutes, 4 days a week.

Pitta/Mesomorph: Alternate between Sun Salutations A, B, and C, practicing for 35 to 40 minutes, 4 days a week.

Kapha/Endomorph: Alternate between Sun Salutations A, B, and C, practicing for 45 to 50 minutes, 5 or 6 days a week.

Warm Up: Perform Sun Salutation A once slowly, holding each posture for 5 breaths.

Sun Salutation:

Vata/Ectomorph: Perform 4 repetitions of Sun Salutation A, or perform Sun Salutation B 3 times, or Sun Salutation C 2 times. Pace yourself at 50 percent of your maximum heart rate (see "Your Heart Rate," page 41).

Pitta/Mesomorph: Perform 5 repetitions of Sun Salutation A, or perform Sun Salutation B 4 times, or Sun Salutation C 3 times. Pace yourself at 55 percent of your maximum heart rate (see "Your Heart Rate," page 41).

Kapha/Endomorph: Perform Sun Salutation A 6 times, or perform Sun Salutation B 5 times, or Sun Salutation C 4 times. Pace yourself at 60 to 65 percent of your maximum heart rate (see "Your Heart Rate," page 41).

Cool Down: Perform 1 repetition of Sun Salutation A slowly, holding each posture for 5 breaths. End with 5 to 10 minutes of Supported Relaxation Pose.

SUN SALUTATION A *(SURYA NAMASKAR VARIATION A):* BEGINNER AND WARM-UP

What It Is: This ancient, classic yoga routine is traditionally done at sunrise, but can of course be practiced anytime during the day. It is a complete workout for body and mind.

1. Mountain Pose *(Tadasana):* Stand with your feet together, legs straight, kneecaps tightened and pulled up, weight distributed evenly, and hands in prayer position over your heart center. Tilt your pelvis under, abdomen pulled in and shoulders relaxed and down, away from your ears. Lift your sternum toward the ceiling.

2. Standing Backbend *(Hasta Uttanasana)*: Inhale and raise your arms in a V overhead. Tighten your buttock muscles firmly to protect your lower back, lift your chest toward the ceiling, and bend backward. Pause for 3 seconds.

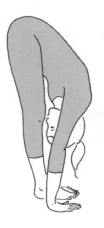

3. Standing Forward Bend *(Uttanasana)*: Exhale, extending your arms forward, and fold your torso forward from the hips, abdomen in. Bend your knees slightly. Relax your face, head, neck, and shoulders toward the floor and lower your chest to your thighs. Place your hands on the floor, fingers in line with your toes.

4. Left Lunge (*Anjaneyasana*): Inhale, bending both knees and keeping your palms flat beside your feet. Step your right foot back, bringing your right knee to the floor. Stretch your chin up toward the ceiling. Your left knee should be directly over your left ankle (i.e., shin perpendicular to the floor).

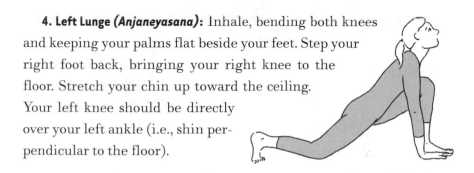

5. Plank Pose (*Dandasana*): Exhale, bringing your left leg back to join your right, and extend your arms, as you would to begin a push-up. Keep your body straight, legs and arms extended and head in line with spine. Pull your stomach in. Hold for 1 or 2 breaths.

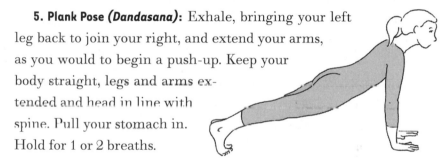

6. Modified Plank Pose (*Modified Chaturanga Dandasana*): Exhale, bending and lowering your knees, chest, and chin to

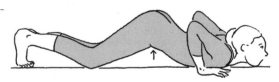

the floor. Hips are up, abdomen is in. This pose is similar to a modified women's push-up. Keep your elbows close to your body. Or, if this is too difficult, go from Plank Pose to placing the body flat, face down on the floor. Then go into a modified women's push-up position.

7. Cobra Pose *(Bhujangasana)*: Inhale, raising forehead, chin, and chest while arching your spine. Hips are on the floor. Elbows should be slightly bent and close to the body. Shoulders are pressed down and away from the ears. Tilt the pelvis under for lower-back protection. Pause for several breaths.

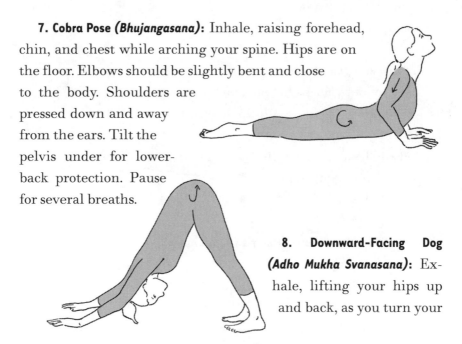

8. Downward-Facing Dog *(Adho Mukha Svanasana)*: Exhale, lifting your hips up and back, as you turn your body into an upside-down V. Keep your arms and legs straight and press your heels to the floor. Shoulders are pressed down and away from the ears.

9. Right Lunge (*Anjaneyasana*): Inhale, lunging your right foot forward between your two hands, toes in line with fingers. Look up, chin raised, palms flat, left knee on the floor.

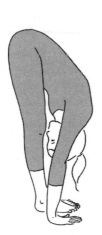

10. Standing Forward Bend (*Uttanasana*): Exhale, pushing off with the toes of your left foot to bring the left foot forward to join the right. Upper body is folded forward from the hips, knees are slightly bent, hands are on either side of the feet.

11. Standing Backbend (*Hasta Uttanasana*): Inhale, raising yourself upright and keeping your back straight, your arms extended overhead, and your knees slightly bent. Exhale and tighten your buttocks. Inhale, keeping your head between your arms; lift the sternum toward the ceiling and arch your spine backward. Pause for 3 seconds.

12. Mountain Pose (*Tadasana*): Exhale, returning to an upright position and bringing your palms together. Take a few breaths, breathing in light and energy, exhaling tension and fatigue.

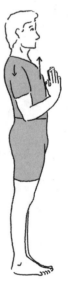

Repeat Steps 2 through 12 on the opposite leg, bringing the left leg back for Step 4, then forward for Step 9, for a complete cycle.

SUN SALUTATION B *(SURYA NAMASKAR VARIATION B)*: BEGINNER–INTERMEDIATE

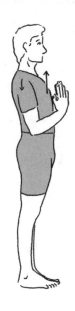

1. Mountain Pose *(Tadasana)*: Stand with your feet together, legs straight, kneecaps tightened and pulled up, weight distributed evenly, and hands in prayer position over your heart center. Tilt your pelvis under, abdomen pulled in and shoulders relaxed and down, away from your ears. Lift your sternum toward the ceiling.

2. Standing Backbend *(Hasta Uttanasana)*: Inhale and raise your arms in a V overhead. Tighten your buttock muscles firmly to protect your lower back, lift your chest toward the ceiling and bend backward. Pause for 3 seconds.

3. Standing Forward Bend (*Uttanasana*): Exhale, extending your arms forward, and fold your torso forward from the hips, abdomen in. Bend your knees slightly. Relax your face, head, neck, and shoulders toward the floor and lower your chest to your thighs. Place your hands on the floor, fingers in line with your toes.

4. Monkey (*Urdhva Mukha Uttanasana*): Inhale, extending your spine from the hips, and lift your head and chest away from your thighs. Roll your shoulders back and bend your knees if you need to.

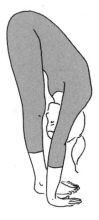

5. Standing Forward Bend (*Uttanasana*): Exhale and fold your torso forward from the hips, abdomen in.

Bend your knees slightly. Relax your face, head, neck, and shoulders toward the floor and lower your chest to your thighs.

6. Plank Pose (*Dandasana*): Exhale. Planting your palms firmly on the mat, bring your right leg back, then your left. Extend your arms as if to begin a push-up. Keep your body straight, legs and arms extended and head in line with spine. Pull your stomach in. Hold for several breaths.

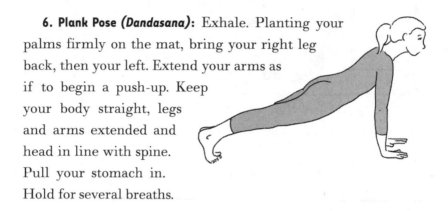

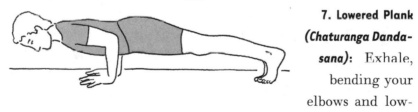

7. Lowered Plank (*Chaturanga Dandasana*): Exhale, bending your elbows and lowering your whole body to a few inches off the floor. Draw your elbows back and close to your sides. Hold for 1 breath, then lower yourself to the floor.

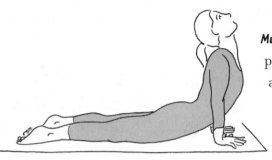

8. Upward-Facing Dog (*Urdhva Mukha Svanasana*): Inhale, pushing up with your arms and chest and arching your back, as in Cobra. Now lift your pelvis and legs slightly off the floor, resting your entire body weight on your hands and the tops of your feet. Draw your torso forward between straight arms and open your chest. Roll your shoulder blades down and keep your buttocks firm to protect your lower back. Abdomen is lifted.

9. Downward-Facing Dog (*Adho Mukha Svanasana*): Exhale, lifting your hips up and back as you turn your body into an upside-down V. Keep your arms and legs straight and press your heels to the floor. Shoulders are pressed down and away from the ears. Hold for 5 breaths.

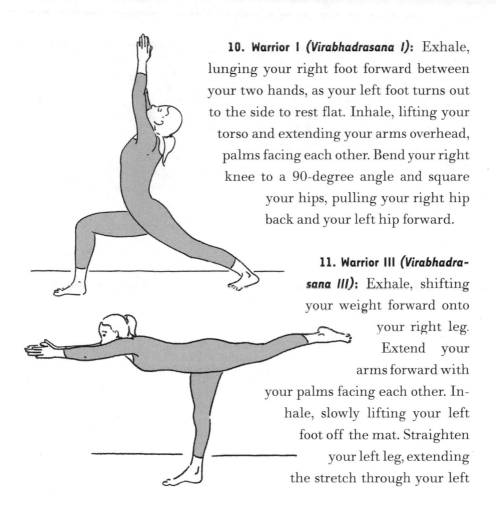

10. Warrior I *(Virabhadrasana I)*: Exhale, lunging your right foot forward between your two hands, as your left foot turns out to the side to rest flat. Inhale, lifting your torso and extending your arms overhead, palms facing each other. Bend your right knee to a 90-degree angle and square your hips, pulling your right hip back and your left hip forward.

11. Warrior III *(Virabhadrasana III)*: Exhale, shifting your weight forward onto your right leg. Extend your arms forward with your palms facing each other. Inhale, slowly lifting your left foot off the mat. Straighten your left leg, extending the stretch through your left foot. Straighten your right leg and keep your right foot rooted to the ground. Gaze at a spot on the floor, but keep your eyes soft.

12. Deep Lunge (*Anjaneyasana Variation 1*):
Exhale, bringing your left foot back to the mat and turning it out to the side to rest flat. Bend your right knee to a 90-degree angle and square your hips, pulling your right hip back and your left hip forward. Clasp your hands behind your back. Inhale, lifting your arms behind you, squeezing your shoulder blades together, and straightening your elbows. Exhale, folding forward from your hips, hands clasped above your head. Bring your face toward your right thigh. Hold for 2 breaths.

13. Plank Pose (*Dandasana*):
Exhale, releasing your hands and bringing your palms down

to the floor on either side of your right foot. Bring your right leg back to join the left and extend your arms, as if to start a push-up. Keep body straight, legs and arms extended and head in line with spine. Pull your abdomen in.

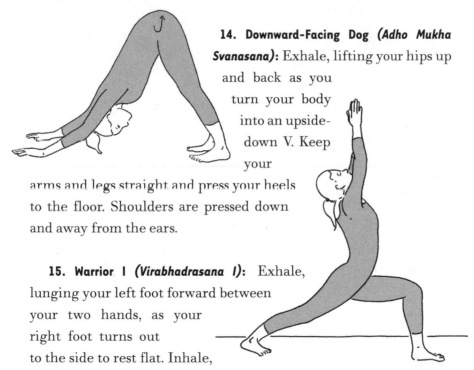

14. Downward-Facing Dog (*Adho Mukha Svanasana*): Exhale, lifting your hips up and back as you turn your body into an upside-down V. Keep your arms and legs straight and press your heels to the floor. Shoulders are pressed down and away from the ears.

15. Warrior 1 (*Virabhadrasana 1*): Exhale, lunging your left foot forward between your two hands, as your right foot turns out to the side to rest flat. Inhale, lifting your torso and extending your arms overhead, palms facing each other. Bend your left knee to a 90-degree angle and square your hips, pulling your left hip back and your right hip forward.

16. Warrior III *(Virabhadrasana III)*: Exhale, shifting your weight forward onto your left leg. Extend your arms forward with your palms facing each other. Inhale, slowly lifting your right foot off the mat. Straighten your right leg, extending the stretch through your right foot. Straighten your left leg and keep your left foot rooted to the ground. Gaze at a spot on the floor, but keep your eyes soft.

17. Deep Lunge (*Anjaneyasana Variation 1*):
Exhale, bringing your right foot back to
the mat and turning it out to the
side to rest flat. Bend your
left knee to a 90-degree
angle and square your hips,
pulling your left hip back and
your right hip forward. Clasp
your hands behind your back.
Inhale, lifting your arms be-
hind you, squeezing your shoulder blades together,
and straightening your elbows, as you expand your
chest. Exhale, folding forward from your hips, hands
clasped above your head. Bring your face toward your
left thigh. Hold for 2 breaths.

18. Standing Forward Bend (*Uttanasana*): Exhale, releasing your hands. Push off with the toes of your right foot
to bring your right foot forward to meet your left. Upper
body is folded forward from the hips, knees are slightly
bent, hands are on either side of the feet.

19. Standing Bow *(Dhanurasana)*: Inhale, raising yourself upright and keeping your back straight. Arms extend overhead and knees are slightly bent. Exhale, bringing your feet hip-distance apart, bending your knees, and placing your palms on the backs of your upper thighs below your buttocks. Tighten your buttocks. Inhale, squeezing your shoulder blades together, lifting your sternum toward the ceiling, and arching your spine backward. Press your hips forward and lean backward as you expand your chest. Exhale and hold.

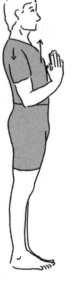

20. Mountain Pose *(Tadasana)*: Inhale, returning to an upright position. Exhale, bringing your feet together and bringing your palms together into prayer position. Take a few breaths, inhaling light and energy, exhaling tension and fatigue.

SUN SALUTATION C
(SURYA NAMASCAR VARIATION C): INTERMEDIATE

1. Mountain Pose (*Tadasana*): Stand with your feet together, legs straight, kneecaps tightened and pulled up, weight distributed evenly, and hands in prayer position over your heart center. Tilt your pelvis under, abdomen pulled in and shoulders relaxed and down, away from your ears. Lift your sternum toward the ceiling.

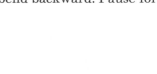

2. Standing Backbend (*Hasta Uttanasana*): Inhale and raise your arms in a V overhead. Tighten your buttock muscles firmly to protect your lower back, lift your chest toward the ceiling, and bend backward. Pause for 3 seconds.

3. Standing Forward Bend (*Uttanasana*): Exhale, extending your arms forward, and fold your torso forward from the hips, abdomen in. Bend your knees slightly. Relax your face, head, neck, and shoulders toward the floor and lower your chest to your thighs. Place your hands on the floor, fingers in line with your toes.

4. Monkey (*Urdhva Mukha Uttanasana*): Inhale, extending your spine from the hips, and lift your head and chest away from your thighs. Roll your shoulders back and bend your knees if you need to.

5. Standing Forward Bend (*Uttanasana*): Exhale and fold your torso forward from the hips, abdomen in. Bend your knees slightly. Relax your face, head, neck, and shoulders toward the floor and lower your chest to your thighs.

6. Raised Runner (*Banarasana*): Inhale, bending both knees and placing your palms flat on the mat on either side of your feet. Step your right foot back, keeping your left leg bent. The right leg is straight, and the ball of the right foot is pressing into the floor.

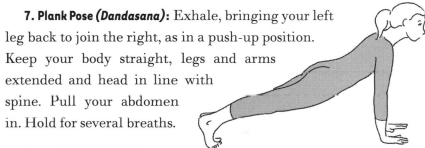

7. Plank Pose (*Dandasana*): Exhale, bringing your left leg back to join the right, as in a push-up position. Keep your body straight, legs and arms extended and head in line with spine. Pull your abdomen in. Hold for several breaths.

8. Lowered Plank (*Chaturanga Dandasana*): Exhale, bend your elbows and lower your whole body to a few inches off the

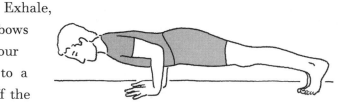

floor. Draw your elbows back and close to your sides. Then lower yourself to the floor.

9. Upward-Facing Dog *(Urdhva Mukha Svanasana)*: Inhale, pushing up with your arms and chest and arching your back, as in Cobra. Now lift your pelvis and legs slightly off the floor, resting your entire body weight on your hands and the tops of your feet. Draw your torso forward between straight arms and open your chest. Roll your shoulder blades down and keep your buttocks firm to protect your lower back. Abdomen is lifted.

10. Downward-Facing Dog *(Adho Mukha Svanasana)*: Exhale, lifting your hips up and back as you turn your body into an upside-down V. Keep your arms and legs straight and press your heels to the floor. Shoulders are pressed down and away from the ears. Hold for 5 breaths.

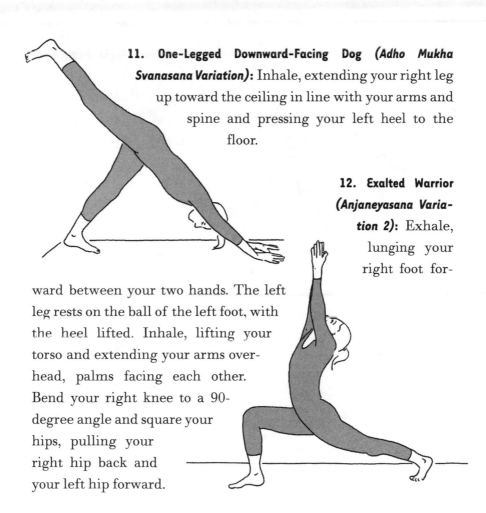

11. One-Legged Downward-Facing Dog (Adho Mukha Svanasana Variation): Inhale, extending your right leg up toward the ceiling in line with your arms and spine and pressing your left heel to the floor.

12. Exalted Warrior (Anjaneyasana Variation 2): Exhale, lunging your right foot forward between your two hands. The left leg rests on the ball of the left foot, with the heel lifted. Inhale, lifting your torso and extending your arms overhead, palms facing each other. Bend your right knee to a 90-degree angle and square your hips, pulling your right hip back and your left hip forward.

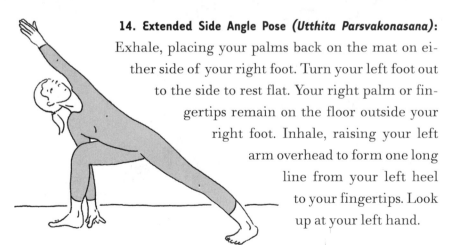

13. Reverse Right Angle Pose (*Parvritta Alanasana*): Exhale, bringing your palms together at your heart center, and twist your shoulders to the right, resting your left upper arm on your right knee. Keep your left leg straight and your left heel lifted. Inhale and look over your right shoulder.

14. Extended Side Angle Pose (*Utthita Parsvakonasana*): Exhale, placing your palms back on the mat on either side of your right foot. Turn your left foot out to the side to rest flat. Your right palm or fingertips remain on the floor outside your right foot. Inhale, raising your left arm overhead to form one long line from your left heel to your fingertips. Look up at your left hand.

15. Plank Pose (Dandasana): Exhale, placing your palms back on the mat on either side of your right foot. Bring your right leg back to join your left, and extend your arms, as if to start a push-up. Keep your body straight, legs and arms extended and head in line with spine. Pull your abdomen in.

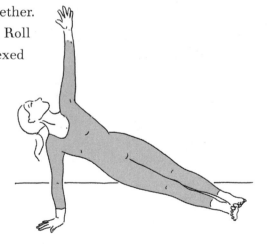

16. Side Plank (Vasisthasana): Inhale, bringing your feet together. Pivot your heels to the right. Roll to the outer edge of your flexed right foot. The legs are straight; the right hand is directly under the right shoulder. Exhale, lifting your left arm up to the ceiling. Look up at your left hand.

17. Plank Pose *(Dandasana)*: Inhale, bringing your left hand back down on the mat, next to your right hand. Both arms are extended, as if to start a push-up. Keep your body straight, legs and arms extended and head in line with spine. Pull your abdomen in.

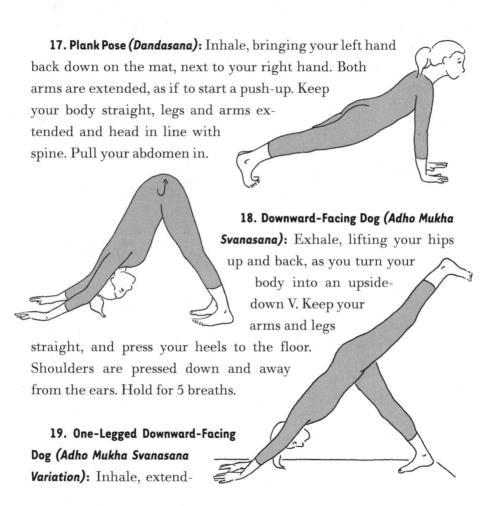

18. Downward-Facing Dog *(Adho Mukha Svanasana)*: Exhale, lifting your hips up and back, as you turn your body into an upside-down V. Keep your arms and legs straight, and press your heels to the floor. Shoulders are pressed down and away from the ears. Hold for 5 breaths.

19. One-Legged Downward-Facing Dog *(Adho Mukha Svanasana Variation)*: Inhale, extending your left leg up toward the ceiling in line with your arms and spine and pressing your right heel to the floor.

20. Exalted Warrior (*Anjaneyasana Variation 2*): Exhale, lunging your left foot forward between your two hands. The right leg rests on the ball of the right foot, with the heel lifted. Inhale, lifting your torso and extending your arms overhead, palms facing each other. Bend your left knee to a 90-degree angle and square your hips, pulling your left hip back and your right hip forward.

21. Reverse Right Angle Pose (*Parvritta Alanasana*): Exhale, bringing your palms together at your heart center, and twist your shoulders to the left, resting your right upper arm on your left knee. Keep your right leg straight and your right heel lifted. Inhale and look over your left shoulder.

22. Extended Side Angle Pose (*Utthita Parsvakonasana*): Exhale, placing your palms back on the mat on either side of your left foot. Turn your right foot out to the side to rest flat. Your left palm or fingertips remain on the floor outside your left foot. Inhale, raising your right arm overhead to form one long line from your right heel to the fingertips. Look up at your right hand.

23. Plank Pose (*Dandasana*): Exhale, placing your palms back on the mat on either side of your left foot. Bring your left leg back to join your right with arms extended, as if to start a push-up.

24. Side Plank (*Vasisthasana*): Inhale, bringing your feet together. Pivot your heels to the left. Roll to the outer edge of your flexed left foot. The legs are straight; the left hand is directly under the left shoulder. Exhale, lifting your right arm up to the ceiling. Look up at your right hand.

25. Plank Pose (*Dandasana*): Inhale, bringing your right hand back down on the mat, next to your left hand. Both arms are extended, as if to start a push-up. Keep your body straight, legs and arms extended and head in line with spine. Pull your abdomen in.

26. Standing Forward Bend (*Uttanasana*): Exhale, pushing off with the toes of your right foot to bring your right foot forward between your hands. Push off with the toes of your left foot to bring your left foot forward to join your right. The upper body is folded forward from the hips, knees slightly bent, hands on either side of the feet. Hold for 5 breaths.

27. Inclined Plane (*Purvottanasana*): Sit on the floor with your legs extended in front of you. Place your palms on the floor 6 to 12 inches behind your hips, your fin- gers pointing away from your feet. (If this is difficult, place your hands with the fingers pointing toward your feet.) Inhale and squeeze your shoulder blades together. Exhale and lift your hips off the floor. Straighten your arms and legs. Tighten your buttocks, squeeze your shoulder blades together, and extend your chest. Push your heels into the floor. Stretch your neck back as far as possible without discomfort. Keep lifting your hips up. Inhale and come back to the seated position.

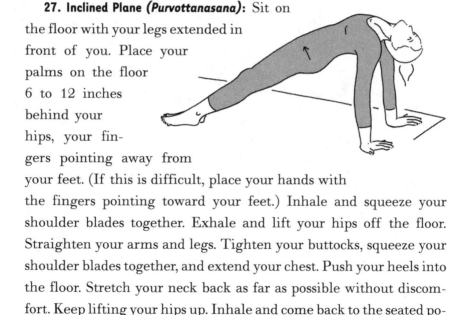

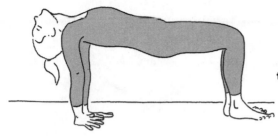

Or try:

Inclined Plane Beginner's Variation (*Purvottanasana Variation 1*):
Sit on the floor with your knees bent at a 90-degree angle and your feet flat on the floor. Place your palms on the floor 6 to 12 inches behind your hips, your fingers pointing toward your feet. Inhale and squeeze your shoulder blades together. Exhale and lift your hips off the floor. Straighten your arms and stretch your neck back as far as possible without discomfort. Keep lifting your hips up. Inhale and come back to the seated position.

Or try:

Inclined Plane Advanced Variation (*Purvottanasana Variation 2*):
Sit on the floor with your legs extended in front of you. Place your palms on the floor 6 to 12 inches behind your hips, your fin-

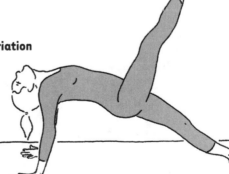

gers pointing away from your feet. Inhale and squeeze your shoulder blades together. Exhale and lift your hips off the floor. Straighten your arms and legs. Tighten your buttocks, squeeze your shoulders blades together, and extend your chest. Push your heels into the floor. Stretch your neck back as far as possible without discomfort. Inhale and raise your right leg. Exhale and lower your right leg. Inhale and raise your left leg. Exhale and lower your left leg. Inhale and come back to the seated position.

28. Standing Forward Bend (*Uttanasana*): Exhale, come to standing, and fold your upper body forward from your hips, knees bent slightly, hands on either side of your feet. Hold for 5 breaths.

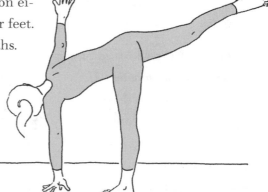

29. Revolving Half Moon (*Ardha Chandrasana Variation*): Exhale, shifting your weight onto your left leg and keeping your hands on either side of your feet. Slowly lift your right foot off the mat. Straighten your right leg, extending the stretch through your right foot. The left leg is straight and the left foot is rooted to the ground. Gaze at a spot on the floor, but keep your eyes soft. Inhale, raising your right arm toward the ceiling.

30. Single-Leg Split (*Urdhva Prasarita Ekapadasana*): Exhale and bring your right hand to the mat. The hands rest on either side of the left foot. Rotate your torso until you are centered and facing your left leg. Keep your right leg raised toward the ceiling. Inhale and continue to straighten your right leg by extending the stretch through your right foot.

31. Side Angle Pose (*Parsvottanasana*): Exhale, bending your left knee and returning your right foot to the mat. Pivot your right foot slightly out to the right. Center your torso so you are facing your left leg and your hands are on either side of your left foot. Square your hips, pulling your left hip back and your right hip forward. Inhale, lifting your torso and straightening your left leg. Exhale, folding forward from your hips, bringing your forehead to your left knee.

32. Standing Forward Bend (*Uttanasana*): Inhale, bringing your right foot forward next to your left foot, with hands on either side of your feet. The upper body is folded forward from the hips; the knees are bent slightly.

33. Revolving Half Moon (*Ardha Chandrasana Variation*): Exhale, shifting your weight onto your right leg and keeping your hands on either side of your feet. Slowly lift your left foot off the mat. Straighten your left leg, extending the stretch through your left foot. The right leg is straight and the right foot is rooted to the ground. Gaze at a spot on the floor, but keep your eyes soft. Inhale, raising your left arm toward the ceiling.

34. Single-Leg Split *(Urdhva Prasarita Ekapadasana)*: Exhale and bring your left hand to the mat. The hands rest on either side of your right foot. Rotate your torso until you are centered and facing your right leg. Keep your left leg raised toward the ceiling. Inhale and continue to straighten your left leg by extending the stretch through your left foot.

35. Side Angle Pose *(Parsvottanasana)*: Exhale, bending your right knee and returning your left foot to the mat. Pivot your left foot slightly out to the left. Center your torso so you are facing your right leg and your hands are on either side of your right foot. Square your hips, pulling your right hip back and your left hip forward. Inhale, lifting your torso and straightening your right leg. Exhale, folding forward from your hips, bringing your forehead to your right knee.

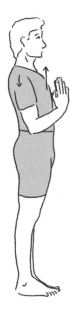

36. Standing Forward Bend (Uttanasana): Inhale, bring your right foot forward between your hands, next to your left foot. The upper body is folded forward from the hips; the knees are bent slightly. Exhale, straightening your legs.

37. Mountain Pose (Tadasana): Inhale, lifting your torso upright, keeping your back straight and extending your arms overhead. Bring your palms together in front of your heart center. Take a few breaths, breathing in light and energy, exhaling tension and fatigue.

Yoga for Strength

Yoga has long been recommended as a way to improve flexibility, balance, and relaxation. What's not as well known is that yoga can build muscle strength. An accomplished yoga practitioner can be as muscularly powerful as a professional athlete or dancer. And because yoga emphasizes strengthening and stretching equally, it is an ideal way to build up your body while improving your flexibility.

The Yoga for Strength Workout that follows combines strength training with yoga poses and includes a customized practice for your body type. This workout will help you create a firm, toned body with muscles that are strong, lean, and long. With steady practice, you will be able to use your muscles more efficiently, avoid injuries, strengthen bones, help prevent osteoporosis, and boost endurance. You'll also improve functional fitness—that is, you'll be better equipped to meet the physical tasks of everyday life, such as picking up your children or your groceries.

Compared to a competitive body builder, an experienced yoga practitioner may be seen as relatively wimpy. Not so. It's true, though, that the type of strength you develop from yoga is different from the type you get from lifting weights. The challenge of a yoga workout is to maintain proper body alignment, activate the appropriate muscles, and breathe deeply while stretching and while holding the poses. I've seen brawny men new to yoga practice shake as they attempted to get into a yoga pose. Often they can't hold the poses at all. However, with practice even the most muscle-bound individual will acquire the necessary agility and stamina to hold these poses.

Poses That Strengthen

Practicing yoga poses such as Dolphin Push-Ups, Pick-Up, Crow Pose, and Plank Pose builds strength by using the body's own weight to provide resistance against gravity. These strengthening poses help build muscle endurance rather than the pure power you develop from weight lifting. You'll become toned, lean, and strong but never bulky, because you're working through a full range of motion using your own body weight as resistance.

It takes flexibility to get into poses such as Modified Extended-Hand-to-Big-Toe Pose and Crow Pose, and it takes focus, balance, and strength to hold them. Balancing poses develop concentrated focus, called *dharana*, one of the eight limbs of the Tree of Yoga described in Patanjali's *Yoga Sutras*. It helps to focus your attention on a single point as you perform these challenging poses.

Practicing poses such as Boat Pose and Boat Pose Variation will help you develop a perfect balance of abdominal strength and tone. By requiring you to move and hold your abdominal muscles as a unit, rather than isolate them as you do when you perform crunches, practicing these poses will give you a long, lean look. Holding poses strengthens all of your abdominal muscles isometrically, thus toning your stomach without compromising flexibility. Practicing yoga will also create a dynamic equilibrium between your abdominals and lower back.

You'll find that doing these yoga strengthening poses will build more than your muscles. The mental focus required to hold these yoga poses also builds equanimity, along with mental and spiritual clarity.

Yoga and Strength Training

At first glance, yoga and strength training may appear to lie on opposite ends of the fitness spectrum, but the truth is they complement each other perfectly. Adding strength training to your yoga workout will develop greater strength, stability, and stamina. This in turn will help you to progress in your yoga practice; you'll be able to progress to more challenging poses.

The addition of free weights to your yoga practice will give you another boost. Doing poses such as Locust Pose with Leg Weights, Chair Pose with Weights, and Side Bend with Weights strengthens your muscles so they become shorter and thicker, protecting you against loss of bone and muscle mass.

Ultimately, practicing yoga without weights will not build as much muscle mass as training with weights. Without weights, the maximum load you carry is limited to your body weight. This may be an issue if you're an intermediate or advanced yoga practitioner. If your muscles have adapted to supporting your body weight, then your regular routine no longer presents a rigorous strength-building challenge.

Weights are also beneficial for beginners who have trouble supporting their body weight in poses such as Plank Pose or Crow Pose. Training with free weights—practicing Biceps Curls with Weights, Triceps Extensions with Weights, and Shoulder Press, for example—can help beginners and advanced practitioners build the strength and stamina necessary to support their own body weight in the more challenging yoga poses.

Yoga Strength Training for Your Body Type

As discussed in Chapter 3, tailoring your yoga practice to your particular body type helps increase your lean muscle mass, energy, and stamina. You'll improve cardiovascular fitness, reduce fat, and achieve your desired physical appearance.

People of all body types will benefit from practicing these strength-training yoga poses, but each body type requires a different level of intensity to create and maintain perfect health and balance of the body, mind, and spirit.

People of a **vata/ectomorph** body type tend to lack strength and muscle tone, so they benefit from strength training with moderate-to-heavier weights for both upper and lower body. While abdominal exercises are important to all the body types, vata/ectomorphs should perform more repetitions of abdominal strengthening poses such as Boat Pose and Boat Pose Variation, since they are more prone to weak abdominals and lower-back injuries.

People of a **pitta/mesomorph** body type tend to be muscular in the upper body with slender legs, so they benefit from strength training with lighter weights for the upper body and moderate weights with more repetitions for the lower body. Pitta/mesomorphs should perform more repetitions of poses that strengthen the lower body, such as Locust Pose with Leg Weights and Chair Pose with Weights.

People of a **kapha/endomorph** body type tend to build muscle and gain weight easily, primarily on the lower body. They benefit from strength training emphasizing light weights and more repetitions for the upper body—practicing Biceps Curls with Weights, Triceps Extensions with Weights, and Shoulder Press, for example—to draw attention away from the heavier lower body. Kapha/endomorphs should use light weights for the lower body, in poses such as Locust Pose with Leg Weights, or no weights at all.

They should also focus on abdominal strengthening poses such as Boat Pose and Boat Pose Variation.

Yoga for Strength Guidelines

Each of us must be aware of our own abilities and limitations. Be sure to observe the following guidelines during your Yoga for Strength Workout.

- Always consult your physician before beginning a new exercise program.
- Begin this yoga workout gradually. It's best to start with light weights. Begin with 1- to 3-pound weights, according to your abilities and limitations. Build up to the recommended weights for your body type.
- As with any exercise program, start slowly and build up gradually. Don't rush or push yourself past your limits, but work gently and steadily to increase your body's capabilities.
- Always move your weights through the largest range of motion possible, but don't hyperextend your joints. Perform the exercises slowly.

- As you advance, increase the weights accordingly to fatigue your target muscles.
- When working with weights be sure to wear proper footwear, to prevent accidental injuries.
- Keep weights stored safely away from children and pets.

Yoga for Strength Workout Plan

If your time is limited, the Yoga for Strength Workout can be practiced on its own. You will reap muscle-building benefits even if you have only 20 minutes to do this yoga practice. For maximum energy and strength, combine this workout with any of the Yoga for Your Body Type Workouts in Chapter 3. For example, see the combination of the Maintenance Yoga for Your Body Type Workout and the Yoga for Strength Workout on page 98.

Be aware that it may take you more than 4 weeks to do this routine comfortably, depending on your physical condition. If you feel comfortable and confident doing the poses in Weeks 1 and 2, proceed to Weeks 3 and 4. Otherwise, stay with Weeks 1 and 2 until you feel strong enough to continue.

Weeks 1 and 2

Practice Schedule:

Vata/Ectomorph: Practice for 20 to 30 minutes, 3 days week, taking a day off between training sessions.

Pitta/Mesomorph: Practice for 15 to 20 minutes, 2 or 3 days a week, taking a day off between training sessions.

Kapha/Endomorph: Practice for 15 minutes, 2 or 3 days a week, taking a day off between training sessions.

Strengthening Poses:

Vata/Ectomorph:

Using light weights (1 to 3 pounds), do 20 repetitions each:

Biceps Curls with Weights

Triceps Extensions with Weights

Shoulder Press

Using light weights (1 to 3 pounds), do 5 repetitions each:

Locust Pose with Leg Weights

Chair Pose with Weights

Side Bend with Weights

Plus:

Boat Pose and Boat Pose Variation: Repeat 3 times.

Modified Extended-Hand-to-Big-Toe Pose

Pitta/Mesomorph:

Using light weights (1 to 3 pounds), do 20 repetitions each:

Biceps Curls with Weights

Triceps Extensions with Weights

Shoulder Press

Using light weights (1 to 3 pounds), do 5 repetitions each:

Locust Pose with Leg Weights

Chair Pose with Weights

Side Bend with Weights

Plus:

Boat Pose and Boat Pose Variation: Repeat 2 times

Modified Extended-Hand-to-Big-Toe Pose

Kapha/Endomorph:

Using light weights (1 to 3 pounds), do 20 repetitions each:

Biceps Curls with Weights

Triceps Extensions with Weights

Shoulder Press

Using no weights, do 3 repetitions each:

Locust Pose

Chair Pose

Side Bend

Plus:

Boat Pose and Boat Pose Variation: repeat 2 times.
Modified Extended-Hand-to-Big-Toe Pose

Weeks 3 and 4

Practice Schedule:

Vata/Ectomorph: Practice for 30 minutes, 3 or 4 days a week, taking a day off between training sessions.

Pitta/Mesomorph: Practice for 20 or 30 minutes, 2 or 3 days a week, taking a day off between training sessions.

Kapha/Endomorph: Practice for 15 or 20 minutes, 2 or 3 days a week, taking a day off between training sessions.

Strengthening Poses:

Vata/Ectomorph:

Using light weights (1 to 3 pounds) or moderate weights (4 to 7 pounds), do 20 to 30 repetitions each:

Biceps Curls with Weights
Triceps Extensions with Weights
Shoulder Press

Using light weights (1 to 3 pounds) or moderate weights (4 to 7 pounds), do 5 to 10 repetitions each:

Locust Pose with Leg Weights

Chair Pose with Weights

Side Bends with Weights

Plus:

Boat Pose and Boat Pose Variation: Repeat 4 or 5 times.

Plus one of the following:

Extended-Hand-to-Big-Toe Pose, with Side and Power-Leg Variations

Pick-Up

Crow Pose

Dolphin Headstand Preparation and Push-Ups: Repeat 2 times.

Pitta/Mesomorph:

Using light weights (1 to 3 pounds), do 20 repetitions each:

Biceps Curls with Weights

Triceps Extensions with Weights

Shoulder Press

Using moderate weights (4 to 7 pounds), do 5 to 10 repetitions each:

Locust Pose with Leg Weights

Chair Pose with Weights

Side Bends with Weights

Plus:

Boat Pose and Boat Pose Variation: Repeat 2 times.

Plus one of the following:

Extended-Hand-to-Big-Toe Pose, with Side and Power-Leg Variations

Pick-Up

Crow Pose

Dolphin Headstand Preparation and Push-Ups

Kapha/Endomorph:

Using moderate weights (4 to 7 pounds), do 20 to 30 repetitions each:

Biceps Curls with Weights

Triceps Extensions with Weights

Shoulder Press

Using no weights or light weights (1 to 3 pounds), do 3 to 5 repetitions each:

Locust Pose with Leg Weights

Chair Pose with Weights

Side Bends with Weights

Plus:

Boat Pose and Boat Pose Variation: repeat 3 times.

Choose 1:

Extended-Hand-to-Big-Toe Pose, with Side and Power Leg Variations

Pick-Up

Crow Pose

Dolphin Headstand Preparation and Push-Ups: Repeat 2 times.

Maintenance Yoga for Your Body Type and Strength Workout

A combination of the Yoga for Strength Workout and the Maintenance Yoga for Your Body Type Workout will help you build and maintain your strength, cardiovascular fitness and flexibility.

Week 1 and Beyond

Practice Schedule:

Vata/Ectomorph: Alternate practice between Sun Salutations A, B, and C, 4 days a week for 30 minutes. On practice days 1, 3, and 5, follow your Sun Salutation practice with the Yoga for Strength Workout.

Pitta/Mesomorph: Alternate practice between Sun Salutations A, B, and C, 4 days a week for 35 to 40 minutes. On practice days 1, 3, and 5, follow your Sun Salutation practice with the Yoga for Strength Workout.

Kapha/Endomorph: Alternate practice between Sun Salutations A, B, and C, 5 or 6 days a week for 45 to 50 minutes. On practice days 1, 3, and 5, follow your Sun Salutation practice with the Yoga for Strength Workout.

Warm Up: Perform Sun Salutation A once slowly, holding each posture for 5 breaths.

Sun Salutation:

Vata/Ectomorph: Perform 4 repetitions of Sun Salutation A, or perform Sun Salutation B 3 times or Sun Salutation C 2 times. Pace yourself at 50 percent of your maximum heart rate (see "Your Heart Rate," page 41).

Pitta/Mesomorph: Perform 5 repetitions of Sun Salutation A, or perform Sun Salutation B 4 times or Sun Salutation C 3 times. Pace yourself at 55 percent of your maximum heart rate (see "Your Heart Rate," page 41).

Kapha/Endomorph: Perform 6 repetitions of Sun Salutation A, or perform Sun Salutation B 5 times or Sun Salutation C 4 times. Pace yourself at 60 to 65 percent of your maximum heart rate (see "Your Heart Rate," page 41).

Strengthening Poses: 15 to 30 minutes of the Yoga for Strength Workout, depending on your body type.

Cool Down: End with 5 to 10 minutes of Supported Relaxation Pose (page 196).

Yoga for Strength Poses

BICEPS CURLS WITH WEIGHTS

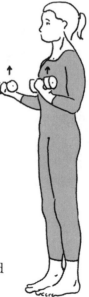

What It Does: Biceps curls work the biceps, the muscles in front of your arms. They help build the upper-body strength and stamina necessary to support your body weight in yoga poses.

How to Do It:

1. Holding dumbbells that are an appropriate weight for you (see the Yoga for Strength Workout Plan), stand with your arms at your sides and your feet hip-width apart.

2. Exhale, slowly lifting the dumbbells toward

your shoulders while keeping your elbows at your waist. Press your shoulder blades down as you lift the dumbbells.

3. Inhale, slowly lowering the dumbbells to your sides. Continue to press your shoulder blades down as you lower the dumbbells.

4. Repeat as prescribed for your body type and fitness level.

TRICEPS EXTENSIONS WITH WEIGHTS

What It Does: Triceps extensions work the triceps, the muscles behind your upper arms. They help build the upper-body strength and stamina necessary to support your body weight in yoga poses.

How to Do It:

1. Lie on your back on the mat, knees bent, with feet flat on the mat, hip-width apart. Holding dumbbells that are an appropriate weight for you (see the Yoga for Strength Workout Plan), bend your elbows and place your hands beside your ears, palms facing each other.

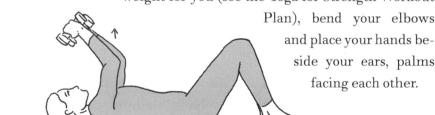

2. Exhale, slowly lifting the dumbbells toward the ceiling until your arms are straight. Keep your arms shoulder-width apart and press your shoulder blades down as you lift the dumbbells.

3. Inhale, slowly lowering the dumbbells back to the bent-elbow position beside your ears. Continue to press your shoulder blades down as you lower the dumbbells.

4. Repeat as prescribed for your body type and fitness level.

SHOULDER PRESS

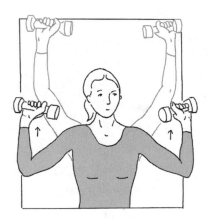

What It Does: Shoulder press works the deltoids, or shoulder muscles. It builds your upper-body strength and the stamina necessary to support your body weight in yoga poses.

How to Do It:

1. Holding dumbbells that are an appropriate weight for you (see the Yoga for Strength Workout Plan), bend your elbows, aligning your hands with your ears. Stand with your feet hip-width apart.

2. Exhale, slowly lifting the dumbbells overhead until your arms are straight. Keep your arms shoulder-width apart and press your shoulder blades down as you lift the dumbbells up.

3. Inhale, slowly lowering the dumbbells back to the bent-elbow position, hands aligned with ears. Continue to press your shoulder blades down as you lower the dumbbells.

4. Repeat as prescribed for your body type and fitness level.

LOCUST POSE WITH LEG WEIGHTS *(SALABHASANA VARIATION)*

What It Does: Using leg weights will supercharge lower-body strengthening. *Individuals with back problems should not practice this pose.*

How to Do It:

1. Wearing ankle weights that are appropriate for you (see the Yoga for Strength Workout Plan), lie face down on the mat with arms stretched down along your sides, palms down, and chin on the floor.

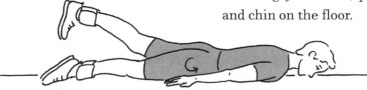

2. Slowly and with control, inhale and raise your left leg, keeping the leg straight. To protect your lower back, pull your abdomen in and tuck your pelvis under, tighten your buttocks, and keep both hips firmly on the mat.

3. Slowly and with control, exhale as you lower your leg to the floor.

4. Repeat with your right leg.

5. Repeat as prescribed for your body type and fitness level.

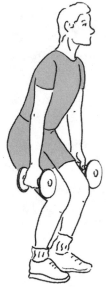

CHAIR POSE WITH WEIGHTS
(*UTKATASANA VARIATION*)

What It Does: The use of weights while doing Chair Pose will supercharge lower-body strengthening.

How to Do It:

1. Holding light dumbbells that are appropriate for you (see the Yoga for Strength Workout Plan), stand with your feet hip-width apart.

2. Inhale, bend your knees, and squat slowly.

Pull your abdomen in and hold your torso erect. Knees are in line with feet. Squat, bringing your thighs as close to horizontal as possible.

3. Exhale, slowly rising to standing.

4. Repeat as prescribed for your body type and fitness level.

SIDE BEND WITH WEIGHTS (NITAMBASANA VARIATION)

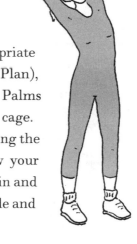

What It Does: The use of weights while doing Side Bends will strengthen the abdominals and trim the waistline.

How to Do It:

1. Holding two dumbbells that are appropriate for you (see the Yoga for Strength Workout Plan), inhale and raise your arms straight overhead. Palms face each other and arms lift up out of the rib cage.

2. Exhale, stretching to the right and keeping the weights an even distance apart. Don't allow your arms to collapse together. Pull your abdomen in and tighten your buttocks. Hold for a breath. Inhale and come back to center.

2. Exhale. Repeat to the left.

3. Repeat as prescribed for your body type and fitness level.

PICK-UP *(TOLASANA)*

What It Does: Pick-Up strengthens the arms, chest, shoulders, and abdominals. It also improves posture by developing superb balance. This is a challenging pose, but as you practice it you will find your balance in the posture.

How to Do It:

1. Sit on the mat in a cross-legged position. Place your hands on the floor by your hips, with fingers comfortably spread.

2. Inhale, shifting your weight forward onto your arms as you lift your legs off the floor, holding them close to your body. Straighten your arms, lift up through the sternum, and press your shoulders down and away from your ears.

3. Continue shifting your weight forward, lifting your legs off the

floor and balancing yourself. All your weight is resting on your hands.

4. Breathe evenly as you stay balanced and focused. Hold for 30 seconds.

CROW POSE *(KAKASANA)*

What It Does: This strengthens the arms, chest, and thighs and stretches the hips and back. It also improves posture by developing superb balance. This is a challenging pose, but as you practice it you will find your balance in the posture.

How to Do It:

1. Squat down, resting your weight on the balls of your feet. Place your hands on the floor between your legs, with your fingers comfortably spread. Bring your knees onto the backs of your arms (your triceps). Shift your weight forward onto your arms as you rise up on your toes. Press your shoulder blades down and squeeze your inner thighs together.

2. Continue shifting your weight forward, lifting your toes off the floor and slowly balancing yourself. All your weight is resting on your hands.

3. Breathe evenly as you stay balanced and focused. Hold for 30 seconds.

DOLPHIN HEADSTAND PREPARATION AND PUSH-UPS
(ARDHA SIRSANA AND VARIATION)

What It Does: This strengthens the entire body, especially the arms, shoulders, and neck. Dolphin is a preparation for the headstand, which requires the supervision of a qualified instructor. Practice this on a mat with a neatly folded blanket or padding for your head. You can still reap headstand benefits by doing this preparation.

How to Do It:

1. Kneel on a mat and then rest your forearms in front of you on the mat,

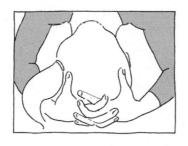

so that your thighs and upper arms are perpendicular to the floor. Measure the distance between your elbows by placing your left fist against your right elbow. Elbows should be shoulder-width apart. Interlace your fingers, forming a triangular base with your forearms. Place the crown of your head on the floor, supporting it with cupped hands.

2. Exhale and lift your hips, straightening your knees, with the balls of your feet pressing into the mat. Press your upper arms and the center of your forearms (the ulna) into the mat to create leverage. Draw your shoulders away from your neck. The top of each wrist is directly over the bottom of the wrist, not tilting in or out.

3. Inhale, push down on your forearms, and lift your head a few

inches off the floor. Exhale and bring the crown of your head back down to the mat. Repeat.

4. As you get stronger, add this variation (otherwise, go directly to step 5): Inhale, push down on your forearms, and lift your head a few inches off the floor. Exhale and lower your chin over your interlaced hands. Repeat twice.

5. Bend your knees and place them on the floor. Keep your head down for a few moments before sitting up.

6. Repeat as prescribed for your body type and fitness level.

MODIFIED EXTENDED-HAND-TO-BIG-TOE POSE (MODIFIED UTTHITA HASTA PADANGUSTHASANA)

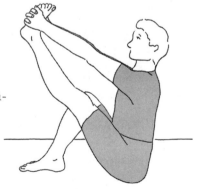

What It Does: This acts as an intense, overall body stretch and strengthener. It is a preparation for Extended-Hand-to-Big-Toe Pose.

How to Do It:

1. Sit with your knees bent in front of you. Feet are hip-width apart and rest flat on the mat. With both hands, grasp the bottom of your left foot.

2. Exhale and extend your left leg out in front of you. Press your shoulders down and away from your ears. Stretch for 2 or 3 breaths.

3. If you're unable to straighten your left leg, place a strap or towel around the ball of your left foot and hold the ends with your left hand. Stretch for 2 or 3 breaths.

4. Repeat on the other side.

EXTENDED-HAND-TO-BIG-TOE POSE, WITH SIDE AND POWER-LEG VARIATIONS (*UTTHITA HASTA PADANGUSTHASANA AND VARIATIONS 1 AND 2*)

What It Does: This intense, overall body toner strengthens the legs and buttocks as it stretches the hips and hamstrings. It also improves posture by helping to develop superb balance. Practice this more advanced posture when you feel comfortable and strong doing Modified Extended-Hand-to-Big-Toe Pose. If necessary, use a wall or chair at first to help you find your balance.

How to Do It:

1. Begin in Mountain Pose (page 25). Raise your right knee and grasp the big toe of your right foot with your right hand. Place your left hand on your left hip and inhale, balancing on your left leg.

2. Exhale and extend your right leg out in front of you, as far as you can. Press your shoulders down and away from your ears. Stretch and balance for 2 or 3 breaths.

3. If you're unable to straighten your right leg, place a strap or towel around the ball of your right foot and hold the ends with your right hand. Keep your left foot rooted to the ground. Gaze at a spot on

the floor, but keep your eyes soft. Stretch and balance for 2 or 3 breaths.

4. As you get stronger, add these variations (otherwise, go directly to step 6): Exhale and slowly draw the right leg to the right. Continue to keep your left foot rooted to the ground. Inhale and look over your left shoulder. Work up to holding for 2 or 3 breaths. Balance and breathe!

5. Inhale, bringing head and right leg forward. Without leaning back, release your hold on your toe, maintaining the height of your leg. Place your right hand at your waist. Straighten your right leg by extending the stretch through your foot. Continue to keep your left foot rooted to the ground. Gaze at a spot on the floor, but keep your eyes soft. Hold the right leg up for 2 or 3 breaths.

6. Exhale, releasing your right leg down. Return to Mountain Pose.

7. Repeat on the other side.

BOAT POSE AND BOAT POSE VARIATION
(NAVASANA AND NAVASANA VARIATION 1)

What It Does: It tones and strengthens the abdominal muscles. *Individuals with back problems should not practice this pose.*

How to Do It:

1. Sit on the floor with your knees bent in front of you hip-width apart and feet flat on the floor. With your hands, hold the backs of your thighs, close to your knees.

2. Lean back, lifting your feet so your calves are parallel to the floor, and balance on your sit bones (the bones you can feel in your buttocks).

3. Inhale; then exhale, extending your legs until they are straight and you are balancing in a V position. Straighten your arms forward, parallel to the floor, palms facing each other. Draw your navel back toward your spine. Use your abdominals to stay balanced and lifted, elongating

your spine. Work up to holding this pose for 30 seconds. Balance and breathe!

4. As you get stronger, add this variation to your practice (otherwise, go directly to step 5): Exhale and slowly lower legs and arms until they're both just an inch or so off the mat. Pause. Don't strain! Inhale and smoothly bring arms and legs back up to Boat Pose.

5. Exhale and bring your feet to the floor.

6. Repeat as prescribed for your body type and fitness level.

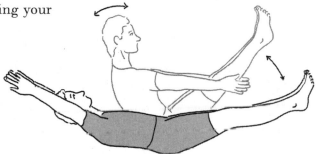

chapter 5

Yoga for Energy

Are you one of the millions of people who feel exhausted on an almost daily basis? Most of us have hit the wall or run out of steam at one time or another. According to experts, fatigue is one of the most common reasons patients visit the doctor.

A 1993 study found that yoga increases physical and mental energy, alertness, and positive state of mind. If you feel your energy level isn't where you'd like it to be, then follow this Yoga for Energy Workout Plan—which includes energy boosting yoga poses and breathing, meditation, and self-massage techniques—to maximize your physical and mental vitality.

Practicing yoga will increase the circulation of prana, life-force energy. The key to high-quality energy and enhanced vitality is the unobstructed flow of prana. By doing this yoga workout, you will accumulate prana and efficiently circulate it throughout your body. With regular practice, you'll build a reservoir of life-force energy from which you can draw during times of need.

Asanas for Energy

Yoga asanas are a sure way to fire up your energy. Stress and other toxic energies are often manifested in tense muscles, which obstruct the flow of prana. Yoga poses release this tension as well as toxin build-up, as they increase the circulation of freshly oxygenated and prana-filled blood throughout the body. Practice vigorous poses such as Yoga Rock and Roll, Woodchopper, and Cat-Cow for an instant pop of energy.

Shallow breathing is a typical response to fatigue and stress; it further decreases our supply of oxygen and energy. By doing poses that open the chest and arch the back, you'll get an extra boost of energy. Try Camel Pose, Bridge Pose, and Chest Expander to energize your mind and body. Follow them with forward bends such as Child's Pose to revitalize and calm your nervous system.

Energize with Pranayama and Meditation

Pranayama is one of the eight essential limbs of yoga described in Patanjali's *Yoga Sutras*. It includes breath control for circulation of prana. In Sanskrit, *yama* means "restraint" or "control." Pranayama seeks to harness and control the breath to direct, circulate, and store prana in the body.

Yoga masters believe that by slowing down the breath, which then slows down the heartbeat, we may enjoy enhanced energy, vitality, and perfect health. They also believe that consistent pranayama practice brings control over the flow of prana in the body.

Doing Gate Pose will help you prepare for pranayama by stretching the sides of the body and the intercostal muscles, the muscles that connect the ribs. You can increase and circulate your prana while soothing your mind and spirit with pranayama exercises such as Prana Breathing, Alternate-Nostril Breathing, Breath of Fire (Bellows Breath), and Complete Breath.

According to yoga breathing principles, lengthening your inhalations and holding them produces an energizing effect on the body and mind. Conversely, lengthening your exhalations and holding them produces a calming effect on the body and mind. Thus we can create a combination of pranayama breathing patterns to energize and calm the mind and body.

For example, an energizing Complete Breath pattern might be a 6-count inhalation, followed by a 4-count hold, a 6-count exhalation, then a 1-count hold. An example of a calming and relaxing Complete Breath pattern is a 4-count inhalation, followed by a 1-count hold, an 8-count exhalation, then a 4-count hold.

With pranayama practice you shift your awareness to your breath, preparing your body and mind for meditation. Yoga breathing and meditation direct your mind away from upsetting thoughts that drain your mental energy. Yoga meditation, such as Yoga Observation, increases your vitality by quieting your mind. It also directs your attention to places where fatigue and tensions have accumulated, blocking your energy. Once you know where these obstructions are, you can release them with yoga energizing poses, so that prana is able to flow more freely.

Beat Fatigue with Yoga Massage

Yoga poses and self-massage are a powerful tension-relieving duo. *Do-in* and self-acupressure are Asian self-massage techniques that help relieve and prevent tension and tightness, promote relaxation, and increase the circulation of prana that energizes mind and body. They also feel great.

Do-in and self-acupressure employ touch, tapping, rubbing, pressure, and stretching to move the vital life-force energies, clear energy blockages, increase circulation, and harmonize the body. Self-massage—specifically pressing and stretching the acupressure points along meridian pathways through which prana flows—balances this vital energy.

For many reasons, such as stress, illness, and aging, tension accumulates around the acupressure points, thereby obstructing prana from flowing properly through the body. Integrating self-massage into yoga poses—Seated Head Tap, Seated Shoulder-and-Arm Tap, Yoga Leg Massage, Yoga Foot Massage, and Modified Child's Pose with Self-Massage—helps to release the tension so that prana circulates freely. This will stimulate self-healing, establish radiant health, relieve and prevent tension and tightness, and increase your overall energy level.

Before You Start

- If you have any physical limitations, such as asthma or heart disease, consult your physician before beginning yoga breathing exercises.
- If you're just beginning a yoga breathing practice, comfortably and gradually work up to the recommended frequency and duration of these pranayama exercises. Respect your own abilities.
- You should never experience strain, dizziness, or shortness of breath while practicing pranayama. If any of these symptoms occur, stop immediately. Try a less challenging yoga breathing exercise. If symptoms persist, see your physician.

Yoga for Energy Workout Plan

If your time is limited, the Yoga for Energy Workout can be practiced on its own. You will reap energizing benefits even if you have only 20 minutes to do this yoga practice. For maximum energy and strength, combine this workout with any of the Yoga for Your Body Type Workouts in Chapter 3. For example, see the combination of the

Maintenance Yoga for Your Body Type Workout and the Yoga for Energy Workout.

Be aware that it may take you more than 4 weeks to do this routine comfortably, depending on your physical condition. If you feel comfortable and confident doing the poses in Weeks 1 and 2, proceed to Weeks 3 and 4. Otherwise, stay with Weeks 1 and 2 until you feel strong enough to continue.

Weeks 1 and 2

Practice Schedule: Practice for 20 to 30 minutes, 3 days a week. Begin with Yoga Massage, proceed to Energizing Poses, and then finish with Yoga Breathing and Meditation.

Yoga Massage—Choose 2 or 3:

Seated Head Tap

Seated Shoulder-and-Arm Tap

Yoga Leg Massage

Yoga Foot Massage

Modified Child's Pose with Self-Massage

Energizing Poses—Choose 3:

Yoga Rock and Roll

Woodchopper

Cat-Cow

Camel Pose

Bridge Pose

Chest Expander

Plus:

Child's Pose

Yoga Breathing and Meditation:

Gate Pose

Prana Breathing

Choose 1:

Complete Breath

Alternate-Nostril Breathing

Breath of Fire

Plus:

Yoga Observation

Weeks 3 and 4

Practice Schedule: Practice for 20 to 30 minutes, 3 days a week. Begin with Yoga Massage, proceed to Energizing Poses, and then finish with Yoga Breathing and Meditation.

Yoga Massage—Choose 2 or 3:

Seated Head Tap

Seated Shoulder-and-Arm Tap

Yoga Leg Massage

Yoga Foot Massage

Modified Child's Pose with Self-Massage

Energizing Poses—Choose 3:

Yoga Rock and Roll

Woodchopper

Cat-Cow

Camel Pose

Bridge Pose

Chest Expander

Plus:

Child's Pose

Yoga Breathing and Meditation:

Gate Pose

Prana Breathing

Choose 1:

Complete Breath

Alternate-Nostril Breathing

Breath of Fire

Plus:

Yoga Observation

Maintenance Yoga for Your Body Type and Energy Workout

A combination of the Yoga for Energy Workout and the Maintenance Yoga for Your Body Type Workout will help you build and maintain your energy, strength, cardiovascular fitness, and flexibility.

Week 1 and Beyond

Practice Schedule:

Vata/Ectomorph: Alternate practice between Sun Salutations A, B, and C, 4 days a week for 30 minutes. On practice days 1, 3, and

5, follow your Sun Salutation practice with the Yoga for Energy Workout.

Pitta/Mesomorph: Alternate practice between Sun Salutations A, B, and C, 4 days a week for 35 to 40 minutes. On practice days 1, 3, and 5, follow your Sun Salutation practice with the Yoga for Energy Workout.

Kapha/Endomorph: Alternate practice between Sun Salutations A, B, and C, 5 or 6 days a week for 45 to 50 minutes. On practice days 1, 3, and 5, follow your Sun Salutation practice with the Yoga for Energy Workout.

Warm Up: Perform Sun Salutation A once slowly, holding each posture for 5 breaths.

Sun Salutation:

Vata/Ectomorph: Perform 4 repetitions of Sun Salutation A, or perform Sun Salutation B 3 times or Sun Salutation C 2 times. Pace yourself at 50 percent of your maximum heart rate (see "Your Heart Rate," page 41).

Pitta/Mesomorph: Perform 5 repetitions of Sun Salutation A, or perform Sun Salutation B 4 times or Sun Salutation C 3 times. Pace yourself at 55 percent of your maximum heart rate (see "Your Heart Rate," page 41).

Kapha/Endomorph: Perform 6 repetitions of Sun Salutation A, or perform Sun Salutation B 5 times or Sun Salutation C 4 times. Pace yourself at 60 to 65 percent of your maximum heart rate (see "Your Heart Rate," page 41).

Energizing Poses: 20 to 30 minutes of the Yoga for Energy Workout.

Cool Down: End with 5 to 10 minutes of Supported Relaxation Pose.

Yoga for Energy Poses

SEATED HEAD TAP

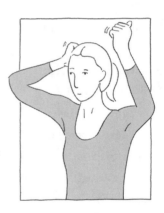

What It Does: Practicing *do-in* in Seated Head Tap helps to relieve tension and tightness in the head and neck, promotes relaxation, and increases the circulation of prana that energizes mind and body. This exercise also helps relieve and prevent tension headaches and improves concentration.

How to Do It:

1. Sit straight in a chair with your legs together and feet flat on the floor.

2. Gently and lightly tap all around your head with loosely closed fists. As you tap, take slow, deep breaths.

3. Tap for approximately 10 seconds.

SEATED SHOULDER-AND-ARM TAP

What It Does: Practicing *do-in* in Seated Shoulder-and-Arm Tap helps to relieve and prevent tension and tightness in the neck, shoulders, and arms and increase the circulation of prana that energizes mind and body.

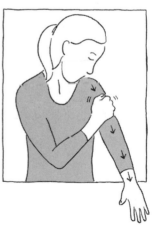

How to Do It:

1. Sit straight in a chair with your legs together and feet flat on the floor.

2. With loosely closed fists, gently and lightly tap from the top of your shoulder, down your arm to your hand.

3. Repeat three times on each arm.

YOGA LEG MASSAGE

What It Does: Practicing *do-in* in Yoga Leg Massage stimulates important acupressure points that revitalize and rejuvenate the body and mind.

How to Do It:

1. Sit comfortably in a cross-legged position on the floor. Raise and bend your left knee, resting your left foot on the mat.

2. Gently press with the index, second, and third fingers of both hands on the outside of your lower left leg below your knee. Gently press from below your knee, down the lower left leg to your ankle.

3. Repeat on your right leg.

YOGA FOOT MASSAGE

What It Does: Practicing *do-in* in Yoga Foot Massage stimulates important acupressure points that revitalize and rejuvenate the body and mind.

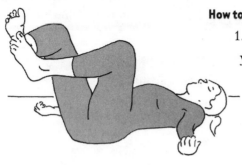

How to Do It:

    1. Lie on your back, arms along your sides, your palms up. Raise and bend your knees.

    2. Briskly rub your feet together, from the toes to the heels of both feet.

MODIFIED CHILD'S POSE WITH SELF-MASSAGE
(MODIFIED SALAMBA BALASANA)

What It Does: Modified Child's Pose with Self-Massage relieves back tension, pain, and fatigue. The addition of *do-in* to this pose increases the circulation of prana that energizes body and mind.

How to Do It:

    1. Kneel in front of a bolster or folded blankets. Place your knees wide apart, with your big toes touching. Put the bolster between your thighs, drawn up to the

groin. If sitting on your ankles is uncomfortable, place a pillow under your ankles and feet.

2. Inhale, then exhale slowly and bend forward, lowering your torso to rest on the bolster. Relax your arms around the support. Turn your face to one side. Relax deeply. Breathe comfortably.

3. Gently tap your lower back and pelvis with lightly closed fists several times.

4. Now relax all efforts. Inhale healing breath into your back. As you exhale, relax your back, visualizing it elongating while releasing all tension and pain. Continue your visualization as you breathe comfortably.

5. Rest for as long as you wish. Return to sitting slowly.

YOGA ROCK AND ROLL

What It Does: Yoga Rock and Roll revitalizes the nervous system and helps eliminate the tensions that drain your energy. Be sure to practice this pose on a rug or a padded mat.

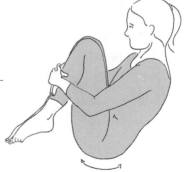

How to Do It:

1. Sit up straight with knees bent and feet flat on the floor. Shift your weight slightly back onto your sit bones, bring your knees to your chest, and give yourself a hug. Slightly round your back.

2. Inhale, then exhale and rock backward on rounded spine, from buttocks to shoulders. Inhale and rock forward, back up to sitting. Repeat the rock and roll 6 times, inhaling as you rock up and exhaling as you rock back.

3. Now rest on your back. Observe the sensations that follow. Do you feel relaxed, with warmth in your back?

WOODCHOPPER

What It Does: Woodchopper revitalizes the nervous system and increases the circulation of prana that energizes body and mind. The vigorous swinging movements of the arms—which mimic the act of chopping wood—give this pose its name.

How to Do It:

1. Stand with your feet hip-width apart and clasp your hands in front of you.

2. Inhaling, lift your arms toward the ceiling. Stretch upward and hold for 3 seconds.

3. Exhaling though your mouth, swing your arms down through your legs (this action is like swinging an ax down to chop wood). Hold for 3 seconds.

4. Inhaling, raise your body back to standing position. Exhale and release your hands.

5. Repeat 2 times.

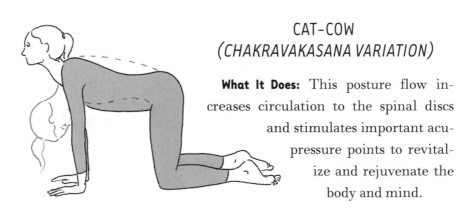

CAT-COW
(CHAKRAVAKASANA VARIATION)

What It Does: This posture flow increases circulation to the spinal discs and stimulates important acupressure points to revitalize and rejuvenate the body and mind.

How to Do It:

1. Kneel with your hands directly below your shoulders and your knees below your hips. Your back should be straight and your palms flat on the floor, your torso like a tabletop.

2. Inhaling, lift your head and drop your abdomen, arching your lower back.

3. In a flowing motion, return to table position as you exhale, then round your back like a cat. Pull your stomach up toward your spine while looking down at the floor. Hold. Release, relaxing your spine and abdomen.

4. Establish a smooth flow of inhaling, lower back arched, and exhaling, back rounded. Repeat 10 times.

CAMEL POSE (USTRASANA)

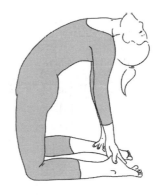

What It Does: Camel Pose revitalizes the nervous system and helps eliminate the tensions that drain your energy. It is an excellent way to stretch and strengthen the front of the thighs and the back.

How to Do It:

1. Kneel on the mat, with knees about 6 inches apart. Place your hands on your lower back with fingers pointing down. To protect your lower back, tighten your buttocks and tuck your pelvis under. Drop your head back comfortably.

2. Inhale and lean back, arching your spine and squeezing your shoulder blades together. If you don't feel ready to continue, stop at this point.

3. Release your right hand from your lower back and grasp your right heel, then release your left hand and grasp your left heel. As you grow more practiced, release both hands and grasp the heels at the same time.

4. Exhale and tighten your buttocks, pressing your pelvis forward. Inhale and lift your chest toward the ceiling. Hold for 2 breaths.

5. To come out of the pose, release your hands from your heels. Leading with your pelvis and using the strength of your thighs, slowly return to kneeling erect.

6. Sit on your heels and relax.

BRIDGE POSE (SETU BANDHASANA)

What It Does: Bridge Pose revitalizes the nervous system and increases the circulation of prana that energizes body and mind.

How to Do It:

1. Lie on your back, arms along your sides, your palms down. Bend both knees and place your feet flat on the floor, hip-width apart.

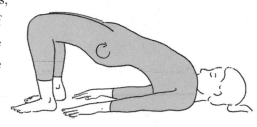

2. Tilt your pelvis, pressing the small of your back gently to the floor. Inhale. Keep the back of your head on the floor. Exhale slowly as you raise your hips up to the middle of the shoulders one vertebra at a time, using your abdominals (building a bridge). Stabilize by pressing down on your heels. Tighten your buttocks and tilt your pelvis under. Hold for 6 seconds.

3. Exhale slowly as you lower your back to the floor, one vertebra at a time.

4. Repeat 3 times.

CHILD'S POSE *(BALASANA)*

What It Does: Child's Pose will revitalize you by calming your nervous system. Follow back-bending poses with this complementary forward-bending pose.

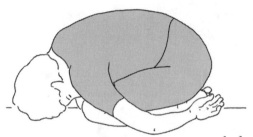

How to Do It:

1. Sit on your heels, with your toes flat and your hands resting on the mat beside your hips, with palms up.

2. Inhale, then exhale slowly and bend forward. Lower your torso and bring your forehead to the floor while keeping your buttocks on your heels.

3. Relax deeply. Breathe comfortably.

4. Rest for as long as you wish. Return to sitting slowly.

GATE POSE *(PARIGHASANA)*

What It Does: The Gate Pose side bend will help you prepare for deep breathing by stretching the intercostal muscles, the muscles that connect the ribs. Use a folded blanket under your supporting knee, if necessary.

How to Do It:

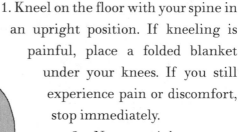

1. Kneel on the floor with your spine in an upright position. If kneeling is painful, place a folded blanket under your knees. If you still experience pain or discomfort, stop immediately.

2. Now straighten your right leg out to the side, with the right foot as flat on the floor as possible and the right knee facing the ceiling. The left knee remains directly below the left hip.

3. Inhale and stretch both arms out to the sides, with palms down. Exhale and reach up with your left arm, then bend at the waist to the right, placing your right hand on your lower right leg. Look up under your left arm toward the ceiling.

4. Hold for 3 to 5 breaths. Stretch and expand the left side of your rib cage with each inhalation and exhalation.

5. Inhale and lift your left arm overhead while bringing your spine back to center. Exhale and stretch both arms out to the sides. Bring your right leg back to kneeling position.

6. Repeat on the other side.

7. Observe the sensation that follows. Does your breathing feel fuller, deeper?

PRANA BREATHING
(PRANAYAMA)

What It Does: Prana Breathing increases prana and relieves stress. It releases tension and stretches the shoulder blades, arms, and hands. It also stimulates acupressure points between the shoulder blades, revitalizing the respiratory, circulatory, and nervous systems.

How to Do It:

1. Stand straight. Inhale slowly through your nose and spread your arms out to your sides. The palms are facing forward. Feel your breath expanding from the center of your chest out

through your arms, to the tips of your fingers. Continue expanding your arms backward, keeping your arms straight, opening your chest, and gently squeezing your shoulder blades together and bringing your head back. Expand the feeling of the breath through your body, down to your toes.

2. Exhale slowly through your nose and bring your arms forward, your palms meeting in front of you as you curve your spine inward and bring your head forward. Bring the expansive feeling back to the center of your chest.

3. Continue Prana Breathing slowly and rhythmically, opening and closing your arms and body with each breath. Continue for 30 to 60 seconds.

COMPLETE BREATH (PRANAYAMA)

What It Does: Research indicates that breathing slowly and deeply sends a message to the body and mind that all is well, thereby interrupting the stress cycle. Practice these calming and energizing breathing patterns to both relax and revitalize yourself.

How to Do It:

1. Sit straight in a chair with your legs together and feet flat on the

floor, or sit on the floor in a cross-legged position such as Easy Pose (page 173). Keep your back straight and your neck and head aligned with your spinal column.

2. Practice Complete Breath with a calming breathing pattern: With your mouth closed, breathe in slowly through your nose to the count of 4. Allow your diaphragm to descend, expanding the middle rib cage, then expanding the base of the lungs. Hold for 1 count.

3. Breathe out through your nose, releasing the air slowly to the count of 8. Exhale from the upper lobes of the lungs, then the middle rib cage. Slightly contract your abdominal muscles and squeeze all the air out of your lungs. Hold for 4 counts.

4. Repeat Complete Breath with an energizing pattern: With your mouth closed, breathe in slowly through your nose to the count of 6. Allow your diaphragm to descend, expanding the middle rib cage, then expanding the base of the lungs. Hold for 4 counts.

5. Breathe out through your nose, releasing the air slowly to the count of 6. Exhale from the upper lobes of your lungs, then your middle rib cage. Slightly contract your abdominal muscles and squeeze all the air out of your lungs. Hold for 1 count.

6. When you finish Complete Breath, sit quietly and observe the sensations that follow. How do you feel? Do you need more energiz-

ing, or calming, or both? Adjust your breathing pattern accordingly. Repeat the energizing and/or calming breathing patterns, depending on your present needs.

ALTERNATE-NOSTRIL BREATHING (NADHI SHODHANA)

What It Does: Alternate-Nostril Breathing, one of the best-known pranayama techniques, helps balance mind, body, and spirit. It revitalizes you by calming your nervous system.

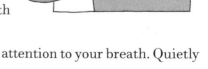

How to Do It:

1. Sit straight in a chair with your legs together and feet flat on the floor, or sit on the floor in a cross-legged position such as Easy Pose (page 173). Keep your back straight and your neck and head aligned with your spinal column.

2. Close your eyes and bring your attention to your breath. Quietly observe the breath for a few moments.

3. Draw the second and third fingers of your right hand to the

center of your palm, then cover your right nostril with your right thumb.

4. Exhale all air from your lungs through your left nostril. Using a Complete Breath inhalation, smoothly inhale through your left nostril, to a total count of 4. Breathe into your belly (count 1); expand your ribs, filling the middle lungs with air (count 2); and bring air up into the upper chest, lifting the breastbone (counts 3 and 4), feeling the base, middle, and upper parts of the lungs completely expanded.

5. Use your right ring finger and thumb to gently pinch both nostrils closed. Hold your breath for the count of 4.

6. Lift the right thumb and, in a smooth stream of breath, exhale slowly through the right nostril to the count of 8: exhale from the upper chest (counts 1 and 2), downward from the ribs and middle lungs (counts 3, 4, and 5), and downward to the base of the lungs, as your belly pulls in with the exhalation (counts 6, 7, and 8).

7. Using a Complete Breath inhalation, smoothly inhale through your right nostril, to a total count of 4. Gently pinch and hold both nostrils closed with your right ring finger and thumb. Hold the breath for the count of 4. Lift the ring finger and, in a smooth stream of breath, exhale slowly through the left nostril to the count of eight. This finishes 1 round of Alternate-Nostril Breathing.

8. Repeat a complete round up to 5 times.

9. When you finish Alternate-Nostril Breathing, sit quietly and observe the sensations that follow. Do you feel calmer, more centered, revitalized?

BREATH OF FIRE, OR BELLOWS BREATH
(BHASTRIKA PRANAYAMA)

What It Does: Like a bellows, which draws in and expels air across heated coals to stoke a fire, *bhastrika* is a heat-generating breath that stokes the circulation of prana in the body. Practice bhastrika on an empty stomach. Bhastrika increases intra-abdominal pressure and should not be practiced by individuals with heart disease, high blood pressure, or digestive disorders, or by women during menstruation or pregnancy.

How to Do It:

1. Sit comfortably in a cross-legged position on the floor. Pull your navel in as you exhale deeply and sharply through pursed lips. Breathe quickly through your nose by forcing air out with sharp, deep, pulling-in movements at the navel. The inhalation is a response to the exhalation.

2. Do 10 exhalations at the rate of 1 breath per second. If the strength of your exhalation begins to weaken, reduce the number of breaths. Build up to 3 rounds of 10 breaths each, and rest as needed between rounds.

3. As you grow stronger, gradually increase to 2 breaths per second and 20 exhalations per round. Repeat up to 3 rounds.

chapter 6

Chakra Yoga

According to yoga philosophy, the body contains seven primary energy centers called chakras that receive, store, and distribute prana, or life-force energy. Physical and emotional problems or imbalances can block your chakras, causing a deficiency of life-force energy in your body. The following chakra yoga workout can open, rebalance, and recharge your chakras so that your prana flows easily, thereby increasing your energy levels and restoring vitality and harmony throughout your entire body.

Chakras aren't just associated with yoga—their existence has been recognized for millennia. Many of the world's cultures, including Native American, Chinese, Japanese, and Hindu, incorporate chakras into their spiritual and healing practices.

In Sanskrit, *chakra* means "wheel," and the seven yogic chakras are spinning energy vortexes located along the spine from its base to the crown of the head. Each chakra relates to a different part of the body and is associated with particular body functions. Practicing yoga poses, mantras, and meditations that correspond to the chakras is better than taking energy vitamins. This Chakra Yoga Workout will help prevent and eliminate chakra energy imbalances and blocks, promoting physical and mental well-being, and increased vitality, and, ultimately, expanding your consciousness.

Energize Your Chakras

You can strengthen any weak areas in your chakras and enhance your energy with corresponding yoga poses, meditations, and mantras. The section "Know Your Chakras" in this chapter describes the location, associated body functions, and characteristics of each chakra, along with signs of deficiencies, as well as the mantras and colors associated with each. If you're experiencing low energy or feeling disempowered, for example, your third chakra may be deficient. Practicing prescribed yoga poses, such as the Pose Dedicated to the Sage Marichi, along with meditation and chanting the mantra, *ram* (see Good Vibrations Meditation, page 174), will open up the chakra and restore vitality.

According to nada yoga, the yoga of sound, a mantra known in Sanskrit as the *bija*, or seed sound, is associated with each of the chakras. Mantra is the practice of repeating sacred words, phrases, or sound vibrations which become the focus of concentration during meditation. Mantras can be chanted, spoken, thought, or written. The sacred sounds of the seed mantras are used to open and clear the energies of the chakras. Seed mantras resonate in specific chakras, energizing and promoting health in body, mind, and spirit.

Each chakra has its own individual color, corresponding to one of the colors of the rainbow. The chakras vibrate at different energy levels, with the lower chakras vibrating more slowly than the higher ones, and this is reflected in their associated colors. For example, the first chakra has a slower vibration than the other chakras, just as its corresponding color, red, has a slower vibration than the other colors. The colors are used in visualization along with meditation and mantra for self-healing, balancing, and revitalizing the part of the body associated with the chakra.

Kundalini Power

The *kundalini* energy (the source of psychospiritual energy) resides at the first chakra, located at the base of the spine. Yoga masters liken kundalini energy to a coiled, sleeping snake, which, when awakened, spirals as it rises up the energy channels (*nadis*) through each chakra, resulting in higher states of awareness and consciousness. When it reaches the crown chakra (located at the top of your head), you achieve *samadhi*, that is, self-realization, pure bliss, or enlightenment.

These yoga poses, meditations, and mantras are designed to open your chakras so that kundalini and prana energy flow freely. By practicing this Chakra Yoga Workout you will gain insight into your personal issues and learn how to raise your energy physically, mentally, and spiritually.

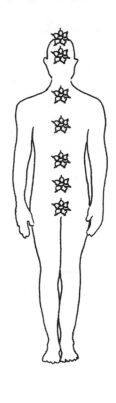

Know Your Chakras

The following are basic descriptions of the seven primary chakras including their locations, associated body systems and functions, characteristics, deficiencies, and related colors. The listings include yoga poses and seed mantras that will open, clear, and energize each chakra.

FIRST: ROOT CHAKRA

Sanskrit Name: *Muladhara* (meaning "root")
Location: Base of the spine and perineum
Body Systems/Functions: Base of the spine, legs, feet, large intestine, adrenal glands
Characteristics: Survival, grounding, security, confidence, self-esteem
Deficiencies: Weak constitution, digestive problems, obesity, fear
Yoga Poses: All poses that bring the base of the spine in contact with the ground, such as Arrow Bal-

ance, and grounding exercises such as Supported Relaxation Pose (page 196)

Mantra: *Lam*

Color: Red

SECOND: SACRAL CHAKRA

Sanskrit Name: *Svadhisthana* (meaning "sweetness")

Location: Lower abdomen, sacrum

Body Systems/Functions: Genitals, ovaries, uterus, prostate, testes, kidney, bladder

Characteristics: Sexuality, emotions, creativity, desire, pleasure

Deficiencies: Sexual and reproductive problems, uterine and bladder disorders

Yoga Poses: All poses that stretch and strengthen the pelvis, such as Pigeon Pose

Mantra: *Vam*

Color: Orange

THIRD: SOLAR PLEXUS CHAKRA

Sanskrit Name: *Manipura* (meaning "lustrous gem")

Location: Solar plexus, abdomen

Body Systems/Functions: Digestive system and glands, metabolism

Characteristics: Will, power, laughter, energy, action, ambition, intention, confidence

Deficiencies: Eating disorders, digestive problems, stress, low energy, low self-esteem, depression, fatigue

Yoga Poses: All poses that strengthen and stretch the abdominals, such as Boat Pose (page 114) and Pose Dedicated to the Sage Marichi (page 167), and poses and vinyasas that energize, such as Sun Salutation (see Maintenance and Chakra Yoga Workout, page 159)

Mantra: *Ram*

Color: Yellow

FOURTH: HEART CHAKRA

Sanskrit Name: *Anahata* (meaning "unstruck")

Location: Heart, chest

Body Systems/Functions: Heart, lungs, thymus, blood, circulatory system

Characteristics: Love, balance, harmony, compassion

Deficiencies: Lung and heart disease, high blood pressure, anger, hostility, loneliness, detachment, overemotionalism, relationship issues

Yoga Poses: All poses that open the chest area, such as Modified Fish Pose, and pranayama breathing techniques such as Complete Breath

Mantra: *Yam*

Color: Green

FIFTH: THROAT CHAKRA

Sanskrit Name: *Visuddha* (meaning "purification")

Location: Throat, neck, jaw, mouth

Body Systems/Functions: Throat, ears, thyroid

Characteristics: Communication, creativity, connection, self-expression

Deficiencies: Thyroid problems, throat ailments, hearing difficulties, neck stiffness, work issues, problems speaking up for yourself and communicating

Yoga Poses: All poses that stretch the neck and throat, such as Crescent Pose, and chanting (see Good Vibrations Meditation, page 174)

Mantra: *Ham*

Color: Sky blue

SIXTH: THIRD EYE CHAKRA

Sanskrit Name: *Ajna* (meaning "to perceive")

Location: Forehead

Body Systems/Functions: Pituitary gland, hypothalamus, pineal gland, eyes, nervous system

Characteristics: Intuition, imagination, visualization, concentration, spirituality, dreaming, psychic nature/higher wisdom

Deficiencies: Headaches, vision problems, learning difficulties, mental fatigue, nightmares

Yoga Poses: Poses that stimulate the third eye, such as Supported Seated Angle Pose, and eye exercises, such as Seated Eye Yoga

Mantra: *So hum*

Color: Indigo

SEVENTH: CROWN CHAKRA

Sanskrit Name: *Sahasrara* (meaning "thousandfold")

Location: Top of the head

Body Systems/Functions: Cerebral cortex, pituitary and pineal glands

Characteristics: Understanding, knowing, thought, spirit, connection with the divine, enlightenment, bliss

Deficiencies: Depression, alienation, confusion, spiritual issues, apathy, materialism, lack of faith

Yoga Poses: Poses that stimulate the crown of the head, such as Rabbit Pose; meditation poses, such as Easy Pose; and meditations, such as Good Vibrations Meditation

Mantra: *Om*

Color: Violet/White

Chakra Yoga Workout Plan

If your time is limited, the Chakra Yoga Workout can be practiced on its own. You will reap energizing benefits even if you have only 20 minutes to do this yoga practice. For maximum energy and strength, combine this workout with any of the Yoga for Your Body Type

Workouts in Chapter 3. For example, see the combination of the Maintenance Yoga for Your Body Type Workout and the Chakra Yoga Workout on page 159.

Be aware that it may take you more than 4 weeks to do this routine comfortably, depending on your physical condition. If you feel comfortable and confident doing the poses in Weeks 1 and 2, proceed to Weeks 3 and 4. Otherwise, stay with Weeks 1 and 2 until you feel strong enough to continue.

Weeks 1 and 2

Practice Schedule: Practice for 20 to 30 minutes, 3 days a week. Begin with Chakra Poses, then proceed to Yoga Meditation and Mantra.

Chakra Poses—Choose 2 or 3 poses to energize, balance, and strengthen your chakras, according to your personal issues (see "Know Your Chakras," above):

Boat Pose
Pigeon Pose
Modified Fish Pose
Crescent Pose
Seated Eye Yoga

Rabbit Pose

Easy Pose

Plus:

Modified Wheel

Knees-to-Chest Pose

Yoga Meditation and Mantra:

Good Vibrations Meditation in Supported Relaxation Pose (see
  page 196)

Weeks 3 and 4

Practice Schedule: Practice for 20 to 30 minutes, 3 days a week.
Begin with Chakra Poses then proceed to Yoga Meditation and
Mantra.

**Chakra Poses—Choose 3 or 4 poses to energize, balance, and strengthen your
chakras, according to your personal issues:**

Boat Pose

Arrow Balance

Pigeon Pose

Pose Dedicated to the Sage Marichi

Modified Fish Pose

Complete Breath

Crescent Pose

Supported Seated Angle Pose

Seated Eye Yoga

Rabbit Pose

Plus:

Wheel Pose

Knees-to-Chest Pose

Yoga Meditation and Mantra:

Good Vibrations Meditation in Easy Pose

Maintenance Yoga for Your Body Type and Chakra Workout

A combination of the Chakra Yoga Workout and the Maintenance Yoga for Your Body Type Workout will help you build and maintain your energy, strength, cardiovascular fitness, and flexibility.

Weeks 1 and Beyond

Practice Schedule:

Vata/Ectomorph: Alternate practice between Sun Salutations A, B, and C, 4 days a week for 30 minutes. On practice days 1, 3, and 5, follow your Sun Salutation practice with the Chakra Yoga Workout.

Pitta/Mesomorph: Alternate practice between Sun Salutations A, B, and C, 4 days a week for 35 to 40 minutes. On practice days 1, 3, and 5, follow your Sun Salutation practice with the Chakra Yoga Workout.

Kapha/Endomorph: Alternate practice between Sun Salutations A, B, and C, 5 or 6 days a week for 45 to 50 minutes. On practice days 1, 3, and 5, follow your Sun Salutation practice with the Chakra Yoga Workout.

Warm Up: Perform Sun Salutation A once slowly, holding each posture for 5 breaths.

Sun Salutation:

Vata/Ectomorph: Perform 4 repetitions of Sun Salutation A, or perform Sun Salutation B 3 times or Sun Salutation C 2 times. Pace yourself at 50 percent of your maximum heart rate (see "Your Heart Rate," page 41).

Pitta/Mesomorph: Perform 5 repetitions of Sun Salutation A, or perform Sun Salutation B 4 times or Sun Salutation C 3 times. Pace yourself at 55 percent of your maximum heart rate (see "Your Heart Rate," page 41).

Kapha/Endomorph: Perform 6 repetitions of Sun Salutation A, or perform Sun Salutation B 5 times or Sun Salutation C 4 times. Pace yourself at 60 to 65 percent of your maximum heart rate (see "Your Heart Rate," page 41).

Chakra Poses: 20 minutes of the Chakra Yoga Workout.

Cool Down: End with 5 to 10 minutes of Supported Relaxation Pose (see page 196).

Chakra Yoga Poses

MODIFIED WHEEL AND WHEEL POSE (MODIFIED CHAKRASANA 1 AND CHAKRASANA)

What It Does: Modified Wheel or Wheel Pose stretches the front of your body and opens all of your chakras. It strengthens your arms and legs, releases tension, revitalizes the nervous system, and increases the circulation of prana that will energize your body and mind. Follow either of these asanas with Knees-to-Chest Pose (page 163).

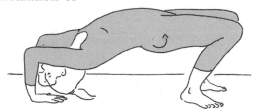

How to Do It:

1. Lie on your back, knees bent, with feet flat

on the mat, hip-width apart. Place your hands palms down under your shoulders, with your fingertips pointing toward your feet.

2. Exhale and tilt your pelvis, pressing the small of your back gently to the floor. Inhale. While slowly exhaling, raise your hips and your back up to the shoulders, one vertebra at a time. Press down on the heels of your hands and push off your shoulders, coming to the top of your head. Stabilize by pressing down on your hands and your heels. Tighten your buttocks and tilt your pelvis under. Hold Modified Wheel for 1 breath.

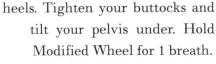

3. When you are strong enough to straighten your arms, continue to Wheel Pose (otherwise, go directly to step 5): Exhaling, press down on the heels of your hands and straighten your arms. Keep your head and neck relaxed as you lift off the floor. Stabilize by pressing down on your hands and your heels. Continue to tighten your buttocks and tilt your pelvis under, lifting your hips toward the ceiling. Pause. Don't strain!

4. As you grow stronger, continue with this pose (otherwise, go directly to step 5): Inhaling, tighten your buttocks and tilt your pelvis under while lifting your hips toward the ceiling. Exhaling, press down on your hands and your heels while pushing your sternum forward toward the wall you are facing. With each of the next 2 inhalations, increase the lifting of the hips, and with each exhalation deepen the stretch of the torso.

5. Exhaling slowly, bend your arms and bring the top of your head to the floor. Then slowly lower your shoulders and spine down to the floor, one vertebra at a time, to the beginning position.

KNEES-TO-CHEST POSE (PAVANAMUKTASANA)

What It Does: Knees-to-Chest Pose stretches the lower-back muscles. Follow Modified Wheel or Wheel Pose with this complementary pose.

How to Do It:

1. Lie on your back, knees bent, with feet flat on the mat, hip-width apart. Bring your knees in to your chest.

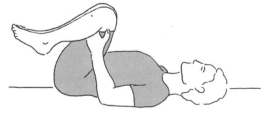

Hold the backs of your thighs and bring your thighs as close to your rib cage as possible.

2. Inhale. Exhale and slowly pull your thighs toward your chest, lifting your buttocks slightly off the floor.

3. Inhale and release your buttocks back down to the floor. Breathe and hold the pose for 30 to 60 seconds.

ARROW BALANCE (NAVASANA VARIATION 2)

What It Does: Arrow Balance energizes the first chakra area, at the base of the spine. It tones and strengthens your abdominal muscles and lower back, while stretching your hamstrings and shoulders. As a balance pose, it also increases your focus and concentration. This is an intermediate pose and should be attempted only when the Boat Pose (page 114) has been mastered.

How to Do It:

1. Sit on the floor with your knees bent in front of you hip-width apart and feet flat on the floor. With your hands, hold the backs of your thighs, close to your knees.

2. Lean back, lifting your feet so your calves are parallel to the floor, and balance on your sit bones (the bones you can feel in your buttocks).

3. Inhale; then exhale, extending your legs until they are straight and you are balancing in a V position. Now raise your legs higher, drawing your chest and thighs closer together. Firmly clasp the soles of your feet with your hands. Raise your head and look up, focusing on a point above you. Draw your navel in toward your spine. Use your abdominals to stay balanced and lifted, elongating your spine. Work up to holding this pose for 3 breaths. As you hold the pose, breathe in and out, silently repeating the mantra *lam* with each inhalation and exhalation.

4. Inhale and bring your feet to the floor.

PIGEON POSE (*EKA PADA RAJAKAPOTASANA*)

What It Does: Pigeon Pose energizes the second chakra area of the pelvis and sacrum. It is a classic hip opener that stretches, aligns, and strengthens the pelvis and sacrum.

How to Do It:

1. Kneel on a mat on your hands and knees. Inhaling, step your left foot forward between your hands into a lunge. Slightly shift the right knee back and rest it on the floor.

2. Exhaling, drop the left knee to the floor between your hands. The left foot should be slightly flexed so that you are putting weight on the outer side of your foot and not on your ankle. Straighten your right leg behind you. Continue to stretch your right leg back, moving your hips as close to the floor as possible. If your left buttock won't reach the floor, support it with a folded blanket. Square your hips and torso, pressing the right hip forward and the outer left hip back. Bring your hands back a little closer to your hips.

4. Inhaling, lift your sternum and arch backward, letting your chest rise like a pigeon's. Press your shoulder blades back and down. Tilt your pelvis under. Hold for up to 3 breaths. As you hold the pose, breathe in and out, silently repeating the mantra *vam* with each inhalation and exhalation.

5. Return to kneeling position. Repeat on the other side.

POSE DEDICATED TO THE SAGE MARICHI
(MARICHYASANA)

What It Does: This pose energizes the third chakra area of the solar plexus and abdomen and the kundalini. As a spinal twist, it also tones the spine and improves digestion and elimination, as it strengthens the back.

How to Do It:

1. Sit with your legs extended in front of you. Inhaling, bend your left knee and bring your left foot over the outside of your right leg. The left foot is flat on the floor.

2. Exhaling, turn your torso to the left. Place your bent right elbow over the outside of your left knee. Place your left hand on the floor by your left hip. Press your shoulders down and away from your ears. Look over your left shoulder.

3. Hold the pose for up to 3 breaths. As you hold the pose, breathe in and out, silently repeating the mantra *ram* with each inhalation and exhalation.

4. Release the twist and return to starting position. Repeat the pose on the other side.

MODIFIED FISH POSE *(MODIFIED MATSYASANA)*

What It Does: Modified Fish Pose energizes the fourth chakra area of the chest. It increases circulation to the thyroid and adrenal glands and lymph nodes, and it improves posture by opening the chest and stretching the upper back. Use a bolster or folded blankets under your back to help stretch and open the chest and upper back.

How to Do It:

1. Sit with your legs extended in front of you and the small of your back a few inches away from the bolster. Then lean against the bolster and arch your back over it. Slowly drop your head back, keeping your arms along your sides. Take 2 deep breaths.

2. Now raise your arms toward the ceiling and gently move them

behind your head, so the backs of your hands touch the floor. Bend your arms if you are stiff and find this action painful. Taking full, deep breaths, hold this pose for up to a minute. As you hold the pose, breathe in and out, silently repeating the mantra *yam* with each inhalation and exhalation.

3. To come out of this pose, roll to one side, then use your arms to help you sit up.

CRESCENT POSE *(ARDHA CHANDRASANA)*

What It Does: Crescent Pose energizes the fifth chakra area of the neck and throat. It increases circulation to your thyroid, and it stretches the neck and throat.

How to Do It:

1. Stand with your legs hip-width apart. With bent arms, clasp your hands (fingers intertwined) together in front of your chest, then extend your index fingers.

2. Inhale as you straighten your arms overhead with your hands clasped together. Exhaling, bend backward from the base of your spine to a 60-degree

angle and drop your head back. Hold the pose for 2 breaths. As you hold the pose, breathe in and out, silently repeating the mantra *ham* with each inhalation and exhalation.

3. Exhale as you return to the starting position.

SEATED EYE YOGA

What It Does: Yoga eye exercises energize the sixth chakra area of the forehead. They will help maintain the strength and health of your eyes as well as prevent eyestrain and tiredness. Do this exercise gradually; do not overtire or strain your eyes.

How to Do It:

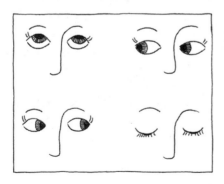

1. Sit comfortably in a chair with feet flat on the floor and shoes off. If you wear eyeglasses, remove them. Circle your eyes slowly in a clockwise direction: raise your eyes up to the ceiling, move them to the right as far as possible, down to the floor, and to

the left as far as possible. There should be no strain or pain while doing this.

2. Repeat the complete circle with your eyes in the opposite—counterclockwise—direction.

3. Work gradually up to 2 repetitions in each direction.

4. Now rest and relax your eyes. Rub your hands together vigorously to warm them. Place your palms lightly over your eyes for a minute. Next, with your fingertips, gently massage around your eyes and along your cheekbones.

SUPPORTED SEATED ANGLE POSE
(SUPPORTED UPAVISTHA KONASANA)

What It Does: This pose energizes the sixth chakra area of the forehead. It also gently opens the legs, hips, and pelvis, while revitalizing the body and mind.

How to Do It:

1. Sit on the floor with a bolster or sev-

eral folded blankets in front of you. Extend your legs and spread them apart. Put the bolster between your thighs, drawn up to the groin.

2. Inhale, then exhale slowly and bend forward, lowering your torso to rest on the bolster. Relax your arms around the support. Rest your forehead on the blankets. Breathe comfortably and rest in the pose for up to 5 minutes. As you hold the pose breathe in and out, silently saying *so* with each inhalation and *hum* with each exhalation.

3. Return to sitting slowly.

RABBIT POSE

What It Does: This pose energizes the seventh chakra area, at the top of the head. It relieves neck tension and increases the circulation to the upper body and to the brain.

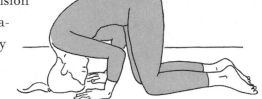

How to Do It:

1. Sit on your heels,

with your toes flat and your hands resting on the mat beside your hips, palms up.

2. Inhale. Exhale slowly and lower your torso, bringing your forehead to the floor while keeping your buttocks on your heels.

3. Place your hands palms down under your shoulders, with your fingertips pointing toward your head. Raise your hips up from your heels and gently move forward as you roll onto the top of your head.

4. Relax and hold the pose for 2 or 3 breaths. As you hold the pose, breathe in and out, silently repeating the mantra *om* with each inhalation and exhalation.

4. Return to sitting slowly.

EASY POSE *(SUKHASANA)*

What It Does: Easy Pose is used for meditations that energize the seventh chakra. It also increases flexibility in the hips, legs, and ankles. Practice this pose with the Good Vibrations Meditation, which follows.

How to Do It:

1. Sit on the floor on the edge of a folded

blanket, to support your hips. Cross your legs. Sit with spine straight. Your knees should be lower than the top of your pelvis. If your back is rounded, or your knees are higher than your pelvis, add another blanket.

2. Place your hands on your knees, palms turned up. Close your eyes and bring your attention to your breath. If you wish, practice Good Vibrations Meditation.

3. As your flexibility increases, dispense with the blanket and sit directly on the floor, centering your weight on your sit bones.

GOOD VIBRATIONS MEDITATION

What It Does: Good Vibrations Meditation energizes, strengthens, unblocks, and balances all the chakras. Focus on any or all of the following chakra meditations according to your personal issues (see "Know Your Chakras," page 151) and available meditation time.

How to Do It:

1. Sit straight in a chair with your legs together and feet flat on the floor; or assume a seated meditation pose, such as Easy Pose, or lie down in Supported Relaxation Pose (page 196). You should be comfortable and relaxed in the position you choose.

2. Close your eyes and bring your attention to your breath. Quietly observe the breath for a few moments. Then, focusing on the first chakra area, at the base of the spine and perineum, visualize a red wheel of light spinning clockwise. As you breathe in, imagine breathing red light into the first chakra. Hold the breath for a moment, imagining that the chakra is absorbing the energy, becoming stronger and healing itself. As you breathe out, chant or silently say to yourself the first chakra mantra, *lam*. Repeat, breathing in the color and breathing out the mantra as often as you wish.

3. Repeat this meditation with each chakra you wish to energize: Focusing on the second chakra area, at the lower abdomen and sacrum, visualize an orange wheel of light spinning clockwise. As you breathe in, imagine breathing orange light into the second chakra. Hold the breath for a moment, imagining that the chakra is absorbing the energy, becoming stronger and healing itself. As you breathe out, chant or silently say to yourself the second chakra mantra, *vam*. Repeat, breathing in the color and breathing out the mantra as often as you wish.

4. Focusing on the third chakra area, at the solar plexus and abdomen, visualize a yellow wheel of light spinning clockwise. As you breathe in, imagine breathing yellow light into the third chakra.

Hold the breath for a moment, imagining that the chakra is absorbing the energy, becoming stronger and healing itself. As you breathe out, chant or silently say to yourself the third chakra mantra, *ram*. Repeat, breathing in the color and breathing out the mantra as often as you wish.

5. Focusing on the fourth chakra area, at the heart and chest, visualize a green wheel of light spinning clockwise. As you breathe in, imagine breathing green light into the fourth chakra. Hold the breath for a moment, imagining that the chakra is absorbing the energy, becoming stronger and healing itself. As you breathe out, chant or silently say to yourself the fourth chakra mantra, *yam*. Repeat, breathing in the color and breathing out the mantra as often as you wish.

6. Focusing on the fifth chakra area, at the neck and throat, visualize a sky blue wheel of light spinning clockwise. As you breathe in, imagine breathing blue light into the fifth chakra. Hold the breath for a moment, imagining that the chakra is absorbing the energy, becoming stronger and healing itself. As you breathe out, chant or silently say to yourself the fifth chakra mantra, *ham*. Repeat, breathing in the color and breathing out the mantra as often as you wish.

7. Focusing on the sixth chakra area, at the forehead, visualize an

indigo wheel of light spinning clockwise. As you breathe in, imagine breathing indigo light into the sixth chakra. Hold the breath for a moment, imagining that the chakra is absorbing the energy, becoming stronger and healing itself. As you breathe out, chant or silently say to yourself the sixth chakra mantra, *so hum*. Repeat, breathing in the color and breathing out the mantra as often as you wish.

8. Focusing on the seventh chakra area, at the top of the head, visualize a violet or white wheel of light spinning clockwise. As you breathe in, imagine breathing violet or white light into the seventh chakra. Hold the breath for a moment, imagining that the chakra is absorbing the energy, becoming stronger and healing itself. As you breathe out, chant or silently say to yourself the seventh chakra mantra, *om*. Repeat, breathing in the color and breathing out the mantra as often as you wish.

Yoga to Relieve Fatigue

Increasing levels of overwork and stress, along with sleep depriva-
tion, lack of exercise, poor diet, and the demands of our nonstop
society, can lead to chronic, profound fatigue. These stressors can
overwhelmingly deplete our physical and mental energy reserves,
and they are linked to the proliferation of bodywide degenerative
syndromes, such as chronic fatigue syndrome, fibromyalgia syndrome, and others.

Try the yoga poses that follow in this chapter to help you heal, revitalize, and strengthen your body, mind, and spirit. Yoga practice
doesn't have to be strenuous for you to derive and enjoy all its benefits. If you are deeply fatigued or recovering from an illness, or you're
an absolute beginner, the Yoga Basics and Relieve-Fatigue routines
described in this chapter will help you to gently build your strength,

stamina, and confidence without injury or strain. This yoga practice will teach you how to work within your fitness capabilities and respect your level of ability, strength, and flexibility. By doing these yoga workouts you can say good-bye to fatigue and say a happy hello to better health.

Yoga Fights Fatigue

Chronic fatigue syndrome (CFS) is characterized by prolonged, debilitating fatigue, which lasts at least six months. There are a multitude of other possible symptoms that can accompany the fatigue, such as muscle and joint pain, weakness, impaired memory or mental concentration, insomnia, and post-exertion fatigue that can last more than 24 hours.

Yoga practice can be an important part of a chronic fatigue treatment program. Studies have shown that even mild exercise, such as the restorative poses included in these yoga routines, can help CFS sufferers regain their strength. Chair yoga poses also gently restore energy and improve circulation, while soothing the nervous system and quieting the mind.

Inversion poses, such as Supported Shoulderstand with Wall and

Legs-up-the-Wall Pose, can help CFS sufferers by increasing blood flow to the brain. Since many CFS patients have neurologically mediated postural hypotension (their blood pressure drops when they're standing), these inversion poses may offer some relief.

Fibromyalgia syndrome (FMS) is a disorder characterized by persistent fatigue accompanied by widespread musculoskeletal pain and stiffness. Other common symptoms include cognitive or memory impairment, numbness and tingling sensations, chronic headaches, and sleep disorder. Since FMS symptoms overlap with those of CFS, many experts now believe that these two syndromes are one and the same. Associated syndromes that may accompany FMS and CFS include irritable bowel syndrome, temperomandibular joint pain dysfunction syndrome, and multiple chemical sensitivity syndrome.

Practicing restorative yoga and chair yoga poses can be beneficial in treating FMS as well as CFS. For FMS (but not CFS), the addition of a regular aerobic practice, such as walking or vinyasa *yoga*, can also help. Research indicates that aerobic exercise is an important nondrug intervention for FMS. To derive the benefits of aerobic exercise, try the Yoga for Your Body Type Workouts found in Chapter 3, once you feel comfortable and confident doing the following Yoga Basics and Relieve-Fatigue Workout.

Chair Yoga

Yoga can be modified for absolute beginners, or for anyone with limited flexibility, tight joints, or other physical challenges. If you have difficulty lying or sitting on the floor, yoga can be done in a chair or on the edge of a bed. You can derive the benefits from many classic yoga poses sitting in a chair or using a chair for support.

Proceed slowly, safely, and with awareness. Work the poses at your comfort level. Don't ever strain or force your body to the point of pain. Remember, the practice of yoga is the antithesis of the no-pain, no-gain approach to working out.

Restorative Yoga

Restorative yoga is the practice of active relaxation to release stress, restore health, replenish vitality, and live in the present moment. The asanas featured in this routine are therapeutic variations of the basic Relaxation Pose (Savasana) combined with yoga breathing (pranayama). Using props, blankets, and bolsters to support the body and help maximize stretch, restorative poses can induce deep states of relaxation, improve sleep and immune function, reduce tension and fatigue, lower blood pressure, and help relieve pain. For example, folded blankets placed beneath the supine body are used for Supported Relaxation Pose and Lying Bound Angle Pose. You can safely assume an inverted position with the support of any wall as shown in Legs-up-the-Wall Pose.

As you progress, grow stronger, and improve with this Yoga Basics and Relieve-Fatigue program, you will naturally want to challenge yourself—and you should—with the routines in Chapters 3, 4, 5, and 6. With steady practice (modifying the poses with props as needed), you will soon feel your body growing stronger and more energized. You will also feel calmer, more self-accepting, and more optimistic.

Yoga-to-Relieve-Fatigue Guidelines

Each of us must be aware of his or her own abilities and limitations. Be sure to observe the following guidelines in your yoga practice to help relieve fatigue and aches and pains.

- If you're suffering from persistent fatigue, it may be due to illness and you should consult your health care practitioner for appropriate treatment. Check with him or her before attempting this program.

- Begin this yoga program gradually. Don't rush or push yourself past your limits, but work gently and steadily to increase your body's capabilities.
- Listen to your body and know the difference between healthy soreness and pain. Stop any exercise if you feel pain.
- You may want to warm up before yoga practice by taking a hot shower or bath and stay warm by doing your yoga poses in a well-heated room. Alternatively, you can dress in warm clothing.

Yoga Basics and Relieve-Fatigue Workout Plan

Begin your first 2 weeks of yoga practice with the following Yoga Relief poses and the Yoga Basics poses described in Chapter 2. Be aware that it may take you more than 2 weeks to do this routine comfortably, depending on your physical condition. If you feel comfortable and confident doing these poses, proceed to the Yoga for Your Body Type Workouts in Chapter 3. Otherwise, stay with Weeks 1 and 2 until you feel strong enough to continue.

Week 1

Practice Schedule: Practice for 30 minutes, 3 or 4 times a week. Warm up with Yoga Basics poses, proceed to Yoga Relief poses, and then cool down with a few more Yoga Basics poses.

Warm Up:

Shoulder Press and Squeeze

Pelvic Tilt

Mountain Pose and Lifting the Sternum

Chest Expander

Yoga Relief:

Seated Forward Hang

Seated Wheel Pose

Seated Side-to-Side

Seated Twist

Seated Leg Lifts

Cool Down:

Root Lock

Ujjayi Breathing

Supported Relaxation Pose and Yoga Observation

Week 2

Practice Schedule: Practice for 30 minutes, 3 or 4 times a week. Warm up with Yoga Basics poses, proceed to Yoga Relief poses and then cool down with a few more Yoga Basics poses.

Warm Up:

Shoulder Press and Squeeze

Pelvic Tilt

Mountain Pose and Lifting the Sternum

Chest Expander

Yoga Relief: Choose either Routine 1 or Routine 2.

Routine 1:

Mountain Pose Variation

Legs-up-the-Wall Pose

Supported Bridge Pose

Modified Child's Pose with Self-Massage

Or

Routine 2:

Mountain Pose Variation

Lying Bound Angle Pose

Supported Shoulderstand with Wall

Modified Fish Pose

Cool Down:

Root Lock

Stomach Lift

Ujjayi Breathing

Supported Relaxation Pose and Yoga Observation

Yoga Relief Poses

SEATED FORWARD HANG (MODIFIED UTTANASANA)

What It Does: It stretches the back, tones the abdominals, calms the nerves, and quiets the mind.

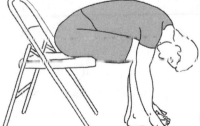

How to Do It:

1. Sit straight in a chair with your legs together and your feet flat on the floor.

2. Inhale. Exhale, rounding your shoulders and relaxing your spine forward, one vertebra at a time. Lower your forehead to your knees, resting your chest on your thighs as your arms hang down by your legs. Feel your back and shoulder muscles stretch as you relax in the position for 3 breaths.

3. Place your hands on your knees and slowly roll up, one vertebra at a time, raising your head last, to an upright seated position. Repeat.

SEATED WHEEL POSE *(MODIFIED CHAKRASANA 2)*

What It Does: It increases spinal flexibility, improves breathing, tones the internal organs, and improves posture.

How to Do It:

1. Sit straight at the edge of your chair with feet flat on the floor, hands resting on the armrests or lightly on the seat of the chair.

2. Inhale and arch, lifting your breastbone. Lift your chin and gaze upward. Do not crunch your neck as you bring your chin up; bring your head back only as far as you can support it. Hold for 3 breaths.

3. Release to a relaxed seated position.

SEATED SIDE-TO-SIDE
(MODIFIED NITAMBASANA)

What It Does: It releases tension and fatigue and tones the upper body.

How to Do It:

1. Sit straight in a chair with your feet flat on the floor. Inhale, raising your arms up beside your ears, your palms facing each other. Stretch your torso and rib cage upward.

2. Exhale, stretching to the left. Pull your abdomen in. Look under your right arm. Come to center. Repeat right.

3. Lower your arms and come to a relaxed seated position.

SEATED TWIST (MODIFIED BHARADVAJASANA)

What It Does: It increases spine and neck flexibility, and it releases tension and fatigue from back muscles.

How to Do It:

1. Sit straight in a chair with your legs together and feet flat on the floor. Inhale, lengthen your spine and place your left hand on your right knee and your right hand on the back of the chair.

2. Exhale and gently twist your body right—turn your belly, then your chest, then your shoulders, then your head, directing your gaze over your right shoulder. Keep your shoulder blades down and in. Hold for 3 breaths.

3. Slowly return to center, beginning with the belly, then the chest, shoulder, head, and eyes.

4. Repeat the twist to the left.

SEATED LEG LIFTS

What It Does: It stretches and strengthens the legs and hips.

How to Do It:

1. Sit straight in a chair with your legs together and your feet flat on the floor. Lightly hold the sides of your chair. Inhale as you extend your right leg

and raise it. Pull the kneecap up so the thigh muscles feel firm. Hold for 4 seconds.

2. Exhale as you lower your right leg to the floor and return to starting position.

3. Repeat with your left leg.

4. Repeat the entire asana once, building up to 5 times.

MOUNTAIN POSE VARIATION
(TADASANA VARIATION)

What It Does: It stretches the upper body and increases the range of motion in the shoulders.

How to Do It:

1. Stand with your feet together, legs straight and arms at your sides, with your palms facing outward.

2. Inhaling, raise your arms out to the sides and then overhead, with your palms facing each other. Exhale. Inhale and stretch your arms, torso, and rib cage further upward, bringing your palms closer to each other. Focus on your breathing.

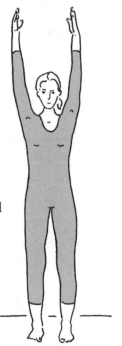

With each of the next 2 inhalations, increase the stretch of the arms and torso.

3. Exhaling, slowly lower your arms to the starting position.

LEGS-UP-THE WALL POSE *(MODIFIED VIPARITA KARANI)*

What It Does: This is a safe and simple way to get all the benefits of an inversion posture. It improves circulation to the upper body and brain and calms the mind.

How to Do It:

1. Sit on the floor beside the wall, with one shoulder as close to the wall as possible. Knees are bent.

2. Swing around and bring both legs up against the wall as you lie back on the floor. Extend your legs straight up the wall with your arms at your sides, keeping your buttocks against the wall. Breathing comfortably, stay in this position for 1 minute.

3. If your hamstring muscles are

stiff and tight, bend your knees a bit. If your lower back, shoulders, and neck are uncomfortable, place a folded blanket or towel beneath them.

4. Come out of the pose by bending your knees, turning to one side, and slowly sitting up.

SUPPORTED BRIDGE POSE *(SUPPORTED SETU BANDHASANA)*

What It Does: Supported Bridge Pose gently opens the chest and upper back, while rejuvenating the body and mind. Use two separate stacks of two or three folded blankets each, or two bolsters, and place them end to end to support the legs, hips, and back. The shoulders, head, and neck should rest comfortably on the floor.

How to Do It:

1. Lie back on the blankets, so that your shoulders, neck, and head are resting comfortably on the floor and your arms are resting by your sides, palms up.

2. Close your eyes and take calm breaths through your nose. Rest in this pose for up to 5 minutes.

3. Come out of the pose by sliding your body backward off the blankets, onto the floor. Roll to your side and pause for a breath or two. Slowly sit up.

LYING BOUND ANGLE POSE
(SUPTA BADDHA KONASANA)

What It Does: Lying Bound Angle Pose promotes circulation to the digestive organs and pelvis, while rejuvenating the body and mind.

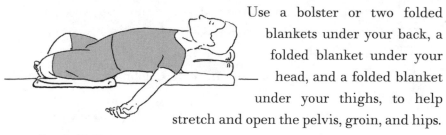

Use a bolster or two folded blankets under your back, a folded blanket under your head, and a folded blanket under your thighs, to help stretch and open the pelvis, groin, and hips.

How to Do It:

1. Sit on floor in front of the blankets, and bring the soles of your feet together. Lie back, keeping the soles touching each other, until your head is resting on the blankets, with your back,

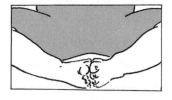

neck, and head fully supported; your arms open; and your hands palms up.

2. Close your eyes; relax your face, throat, and groin; and take calm breaths through your nose. Rest in this pose for up to 5 minutes.

SUPPORTED SHOULDERSTAND WITH WALL
(SUPPORTED SARVANGASANA)

What It Does: This simpler, supported version of the full shoulderstand, known as the Queen of Asanas, will gently tone and strengthen the entire body. Practice on a neatly folded blanket placed about 6 inches away from the wall. Always follow this posture with Fish Pose (see Modified Fish Pose, page 168).

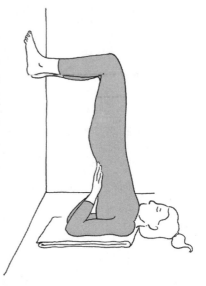

How to Do It:

1. Sit on the folded blanket, with one shoulder as close to the wall as possible and knees bent.

2. Swing around and bring both legs up the wall, lying flat on your back with your shoulders on the blanket. Extend your legs straight up the wall, keeping your buttocks close to the wall.

3. Press the soles of your feet against the wall, bend your knees, and raise your buttocks off the floor, bringing yourself onto your shoulders. Bend your elbows and slide your hands up to your hips.

4. Open your chest by extending your elbows back toward the wall, keeping them parallel to each other. Breathing comfortably, stay in this position for 30 to 60 seconds.

5. Come out of the pose by bringing your hips down the wall slowly and with control to the blanket, turning to the side, and sitting up.

SUPPORTED RELAXATION POSE
(SUPPORTED SAVASANA)

What It Does: This is the granddaddy of all the restorative poses. Savasana enhances the effectiveness of all the poses, calms the mind and nervous system, and helps relieve back tension. End your yoga practice with this pose.

How to Do It:

1. Lie on your back on a mat on the floor with a folded blanket under your head and neck. You may want to put an additional folded blanket or two under your back and/or cover your eyes with an eye pillow or face cloth.

2. Place your feet a comfortable distance apart. Rest your hands at your sides, palms turned upward. Move your shoulders down and away from your ears, and tuck your shoulder blades in toward your spine. If your back feels uncomfortable with your legs straight, bend your knees as much as you need to, to alleviate pain or discomfort. You may feel more comfortable with a folded blanket or pillow beneath your knees.

3. Inhale; exhale, contracting the buttock muscles and pressing the curve out of your lower back. Release and relax completely.

4. Continue to breathe comfortably. With each exhalation, allow the weight of your bones to sink to-

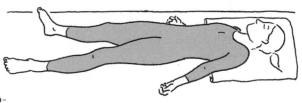

ward the floor. Scan your body, including your spine and your lower back, noting any unnecessary muscular tension. Now, with each exhalation, surrender your muscles to the pull of gravity, sinking further into the floor.

5. Practice Yoga Observation (page 31).

6. Relax all efforts and rest in the healing stillness for as long as you wish. When you're ready to come out of the pose, roll onto one side and use your arms to push yourself up into a seated position.

Index

Single-Leg Split, 81, 83
so hum, 155, 172, 177
solar plexus chakra, 153, 167, 175–76
squeeze, hold, and release actions, 20, 25, 27
stamina:
    body types and, 33, 89
    and Yoga for Strength Workouts, 85–87, 89, 100, 102
    Yoga Relief poses and, 180
Standing Backbend, 10, 26, 52, 56–57, 67
Standing Bow, 26, 66
Standing Forward Bend, 10, 52, 55, 58–59, 65, 68, 77–78, 80, 82, 84
sternum:
    Chakra Yoga Workouts and, 163, 166
    and Yoga Basics and Relieve-Fatigue Workouts, 21–23, 25–28, 185–86
    and Yoga for Energy Workouts, 144
    and Yoga for Strength Workouts, 106
    and Yoga for Your Body Type Workouts, 52, 56–57, 66–67
Stomach Lift, 21, 24, 30–31, 187
strength, strength training:
    goals for, 18–20
    yoga and, 88–91
    see also muscle, muscles, muscular strength
stress, 4–5
    Chakra Yoga Workouts and, 153
    and Yoga Basics and Relieve-Fatigue Workouts, 20, 25, 27, 179
    and Yoga for Energy Workouts, 118, 121, 140–41

Sun Salutations, 21, 28, 153
    A, 12–14, 44–56, 98–100, 126–28, 159–60
    B, 12–14, 46–51, 57–66, 98–100, 126–28, 159–60
    for body types, 12–14, 33, 39–40, 42–84, 98–100, 126–28, 159–61
    C, 12, 14, 49–51, 67–84, 98–100, 126–28, 159–60
Supported Bridge Pose, 24, 186, 193–94
Supported Relaxation Pose, 21, 23–24, 31, 46–47, 49, 51, 100, 128, 152, 161, 183, 185, 187, 196–98
    Good Vibrations Meditation in, 158, 174
Supported Seated Angle Pose, 155, 159, 171–72
Supported Shoulderstand with Wall, 18, 24, 180–81, 186, 195–96

tantra yoga, 4, 7
third eye chakra, 155, 170–71, 176–77
throat chakra, 154–55, 169, 176
thyroid, thyroid problems, 154, 168–69
Transcendental Meditation (TM), 7
Tree of Yoga, 8–9, 87
Triceps Extensions with Weights, 89–90, 93–97, 101–2
Twist, Seated, 23, 185, 189–90
    Left, 10
    Right, 10

uddiyana banda, 21
Ujjayi Breathing, 21, 23–24, 28–29, 44, 185, 187

About the Author

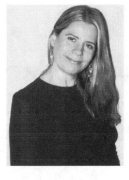

ELAINE GAVALAS received her master's degree from Columbia University, in New York. She's an exercise physiologist, health expert, and weight management specialist who works with groups and with individuals of all sizes, shapes, and ages to help them reach and maintain their ideal weight, wellness, and fitness goals. She utilizes yoga and fitness techniques that integrate the body, mind, and spirit.

Her yoga minibook series includes *The Yoga Minibook for Weight Loss, The Yoga Minibook for Stress Relief, The Yoga Minibook for Longevity*, and *The Yoga Minibook for Energy and Strength*. Gavalas is also the author of numerous yoga, fitness, and diet articles and books, including *Secrets of Fat-Free Greek Cooking* (1998).

If you or your company would like to contact Elaine or want more information about her books, yoga videos, or group and individual services, visit her website at www.yogaminibooks.com or e-mail her at AskElaineG@aol.com.

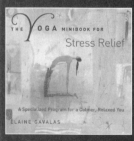
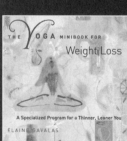
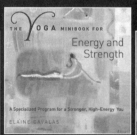
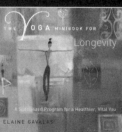